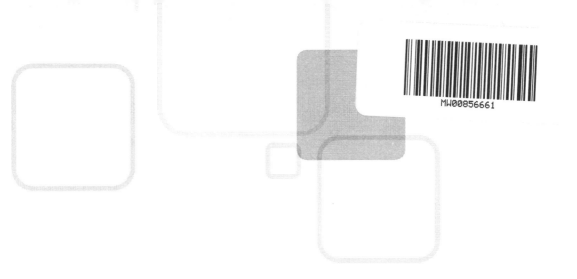

INSIDER'S GUIDE TO THE

ACGME INSTITUTIONAL REVIEW

JOSEPHINE R. FOWLER, MD, MS, FAAFP

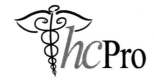

Josephine R. Fowler, MD, MS, FAAFP, Author
Claudia Hoffacker, Editor
Erin Callahan, Executive Editor
Bob Croce, Group Publisher
Shane Katz, Cover Designer
Janell Lukac, Layout Artist
Michael Roberto, Layout Artist

Audrey Doyle, Copyeditor
Liza Banks, Proofreader
Darren Kelly, Books Production Supervisor
Susan Darbyshire, Art Director
Claire Cloutier, Production Manager
Jean St. Pierre, Director of Operations

Advice given is general. Readers should consult professional counsel for specific legal, ethical, or clinical questions.

Arrangements can be made for quantity discounts. For more information, contact:

HCPro, Inc.
P.O. Box 1168
Marblehead, MA 01945
Telephone: 800/650-6787 or 781/639-1872
E-mail: *customerservice@hcpro.com*

Visit HCPro at its World Wide Web sites:
www.hcpro.com and *www.hcmarketplace.com*

CONTENTS

ABOUT THE AUTHOR

Josephine Fowler, MD, MS, FAAFP

Dr. Fowler currently serves as vice president of academic affairs/chief academic officer at John Peter Smith (JPS) Health Network in Fort Worth, TX. She oversees the department of academic affairs, including the office of research and scholarly activity, graduate medical education, and undergraduate medical education JPS serves as training site for more than 180 residents and fellows and more than 500 medical students and physician assistant rotations.

Dr. Fowler comes to JPS from Boston University where she was faculty in family medicine and director of maternal child health (MCH) for seven years. While at Boston University she was appointed associate medical director of MCH for Boston HealthNet Plan, the major insurer of the medically underserved in the Boston area. Dr. Fowler was also adjunct associate professor at Boston University in the Department of Family Medicine and director of maternal and child health, School of Public Health.

INTRODUCTION

The Accreditation Council for Graduate Medical Education (ACGME) is a private nonprofit organization that accredits graduate medical training programs in the United States.[1] The purpose of the organization is to improve and ensure the quality of graduate medical education (GME). The ACGME hosts 27 specialty specific residency review committees (RRCs) composed of volunteer peer reviewers who are appointed by the AMA Council on Medical Education and subsequently approved by the ACGME executive committee and board of directors.

The ACGME is not designed to be punitive toward medical education or training programs, but rather to ensure the training of quality physicians to meet the healthcare needs of the United States. The accrediting organization evaluates not only the educational process of a program, but also the program's ability to make changes in response to:

- ACGME evaluations

- Reduced funding for medical education

- Resident feedback

- Self-evaluations of the program's leaders and institution

The ACGME monitors GME programs and sponsoring institutions in three primary ways, which include:

- **Program accreditation reviews:** These reviews occur every one to five years, depending on the most recent review and the program's assessed compliance with accreditation requirements. These reviews, which include a site visit, focus on the individual GME program and its compliance with ACGME and RRC requirements.

- **Institutional accreditation reviews:** These reviews occur on a two- to five-year cycle. They focus on the sponsoring institution and its compliance with the ACGME institutional requirements. The process includes a confirmatory site visit to review previously submitted information that describes the institution's compliance with ACGME requirements. During the review, surveyors will tour the facility and speak with representatives from GME programs, administrators, and residents. Surveyors will also review documents related to medical education within the sponsoring institution and applicable agreements with participating institutions.

- **Resident online surveys:** Resident surveys serve to verify program and institution function and compliance with guidelines and rules.

ABOUT THIS BOOK

This book will focus on the details of preparing for the institutional review. It will give suggestions on how to optimize preparations through ongoing evaluations and implementation during program site visits, internal reviews, and resident online survey responses.

Chapter 1 reviews the structure and responsibilities of the graduate medical education committee (GMEC). It reviews the key members of the GMEC and gives examples of voting members and nonvoting members. It provides guidance on how the sponsoring institution can collaborate with GME leaders, faculty, residents, and staff in planning for institutional and program reviews.

Chapter 2 focuses on identifying resources within the institution and the roles and responsibilities of institutional leaders and staff. It addresses key policies that are necessary for maintaining resident governance and the safety of residents and patients.

Chapter 3 outlines the sponsoring institution's responsibilities to the residents. It covers eligibility, selection, and appointment of residents. In addition, it outlines the support the sponsoring institution must provide to residents, including financial support and a safe work environment.

Chapter 4 reviews affiliation agreements the sponsoring institution must have with major participating institutions and programs granting rotations to residents. It outlines the required components of the agreement terms for both the master affiliation agreement and the program agreement.

Chapter 5 focuses on the process of preparing for the internal review and the report. The sponsoring institution must conduct an internal review in the middle of its accreditation cycle.

Chapter 6 outlines the steps to completing the institutional review document and some tips on making the institutional review a smooth process.

ENDNOTES

1. Saultz, J.W., and Hill, C.E. 1999. "Lessons learned from *ACGME.*" *Fam Med* 31 (9): 652–5.

PREPARING FOR AN INSTITUTIONAL REVIEW

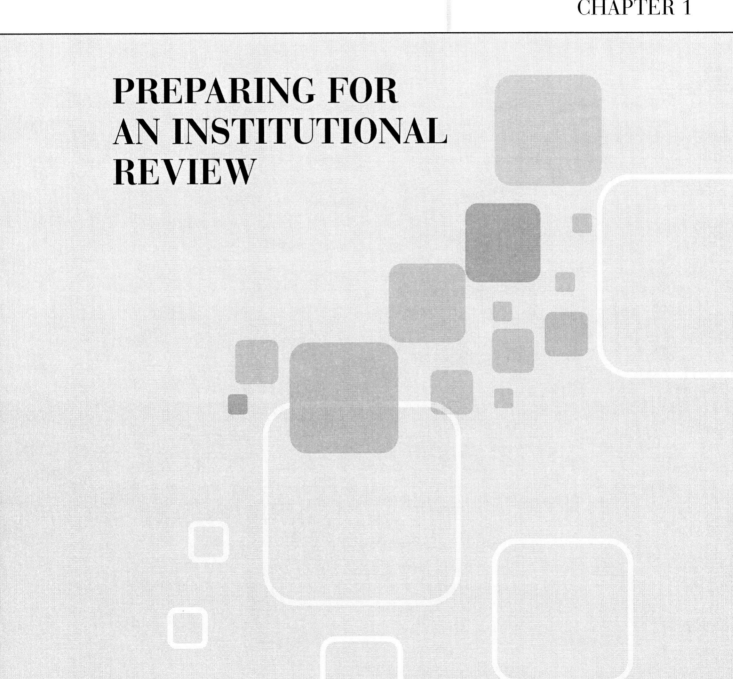

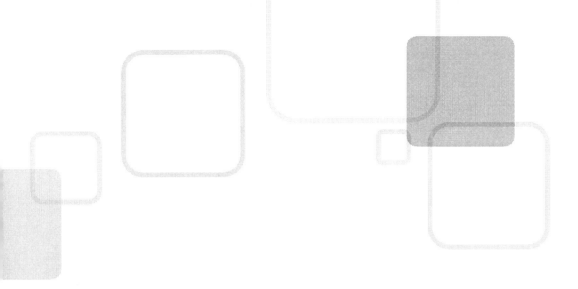

PREPARING FOR AN INSTITUTIONAL REVIEW

As your institution prepares for its Accreditation Council for Graduate Medical Education (ACGME) review, it's important to make sure all the key players are in place and that they understand their roles and responsibilities.

The key players here are the program directors, the designated institutional official (DIO), and members of the graduate medical education committee (GMEC). Once these players are in place, they need to reach out to others in the institution. They need to communicate with others about the institutional review, train them on their roles in the process, and collaborate with them to ensure success.

ROLES AND RESPONSIBILITIES

Understanding roles and responsibilities is paramount to developing a well-functioning graduate medical education (GME) office. The sponsoring institution must commit to identifying capable leaders to oversee medical education and comply with policies and guidelines. These leaders must guide the department, its divisions, and its committees, and provide quality training on regulatory issues of accrediting agencies, guidelines and policies, and updates on plans for improvement of education.

Each organization must identify the leadership that is needed to carry out its mission and strategic plan for advancing medical education. These plans might include a combination of strategic plans from the organizations, systems, and entities involved in supporting medical education in your organization and ensuring its success. (See examples of self-assessment questions for evaluating GME reporting lines and functions in Figure 1.1.)

FIGURE 1.1

Questions to ask when assessing your GME program

1. Who is the primary sponsor for the ACGME accredited programs? List all programs and the sponsoring institution. (Each GME program must operate under one sponsoring institution.)

2. What is the mission of the accrediting agency and other leading medical bodies for GME? (Review mission statements of the AMA, ACGME, Association of American Medical Colleges, etc.)

3. What are the recommendations and guidelines for the sponsoring institution from agencies such as The Joint Commission, Centers for Medicare & Medicaid Services, and Office of Inspector General in regard to training students in GME and regulations concerning supervision, compliance, and sanctions?

4. How can we develop a mission statement for GME that incorporates the strategic plans of the sponsoring institution, the accrediting agencies, while maintaining an overall mission to produce quality healthcare leaders for the physician workforce?

5. Who are the key leaders in the sponsoring institution who champion and support GME?

6. What important information and processes are necessary to report to the leadership of the sponsoring institution and participating organizations that will substantiate the importance of their role in accreditation and financial support? How often will this information be reported?

7. What is the reporting structure in your organization? (For example, do you have an organizational chart?)

The following steps are essential to identifying roles and responsibilities:

1. **Identify all of the institutional partners that are core to the success of GME in your facility.** The CEO and the institution's board members are responsible for the sponsoring institution's strategic plan and play major roles in determining funds and resources

---

committed to medical education within the institution. Other institutional partners include clinical faculty committed to assisting with teaching and research, the chief financial officer, the medical staff and its leaders, ancillary service providers within the institution, nursing leaders and staff, and key administrative leaders that will help to negotiate for space, technology, and resources.

2. **Review the recommendations of key national organizations and governing bodies that are pertinent to maintaining an accredited GME program.** The American Association of Medical Colleges, the AMA, and the ACGME are all focused on improving quality in medical education and patient care.

3. **Establish strategic plans and mission statements that are in line with national, regional, institutional, and local needs.** Creating a commitment or mission statement that is in line with the global mission for the advancement of medical education ensures sustainability within the sponsoring institution and the community.

4. **Identify key personnel to perform tasks and set clear roles for all parties, including the institution's responsibilities and commitment to education.** It is very important to select a DIO and academic leaders that are committed to the advancement of GME within the institution. These leaders are responsible for understanding the interconnection between the sponsoring institution and its academic affiliates and participating institutions. They must be familiar with policies and procedures within the institution and procedures that are necessary to maintain GME quality within the organization.

   The institutional review requirements, institutional review document (IRD), common program requirements, and program-specific requirements can be used as road maps to develop roles for personnel involved in GME. (You can access these documents on the ACGME Web site at *www.acgme.org.*)

5. **Develop a mechanism to inform partners and sponsoring institution leaders of changes related to GME reporting, function, and maintenance.** The DIO and GME leaders may already be appointed to several committees within the sponsoring institution. Meetings are an ideal opportunity to present updates related to GME and the institutional review. Information that is important to accreditation and resident safety, as well as information regarding GME changes, can be presented in newsletters, sent to participating institutions by mail, or presented at a forum for the GME partners.

The GMEC

The ACGME requires each GME sponsoring institution to create a GMEC, which must meet at least quarterly. The GMEC must ensure that its institution maintains structured GME programs that comply with the requirements of accrediting agencies and governing bodies. Each organization must develop distinct guidelines, function, and reporting lines that are specific to its institution and GMEC.

The most important factor in developing the GMEC is to include key leaders in medical education who are familiar with the procedures and guidelines of accrediting agencies. The membership of the GMEC may consist of a chair, vice chair, administrative representative(s), and representatives from all GME programs. The ACGME requires at a minimum the following members:

- The DIO

- Resident program directors

- Representatives from administration and the residency programs

- Resident members

Other members may be invited on an ad hoc basis or as nonvoting members.

The GMEC serves as a peer committee that works collaboratively to monitor program compliance, the adequacy of institutional support, and the quality of educational programs. Additionally, the GMEC facilitates the residents' ethical, professional, and personal development while ensuring safe and appropriate care for patients. Specific roles of committee members are outlined in the upcoming bulleted list.

Members of the GMEC are appointed by the vice president of academic affairs, dean of GME, dean of the school of medicine, chief academic officer, or a similarly appointed institutional official. The terms of appointment may range from one to three years for all members of the committee, except the resident member, who usually serves only one year. However, the GMEC determines the duration of membership.

The following outlines the responsibilities of key GMEC members:

- **Chair:** The chair serves as the public face for the GMEC, and ensures that the committee appropriately complies with ACGME requirements for GMEC structure and function. The chair is responsible for scheduling meetings and notifying members of the place and date of the meetings. This person ensures that each meeting is recorded and prepared for review at the subsequent GMEC meeting. He or she is responsible for appointing subcommittees and delegating responsibilities to committee members. The chair serves as the team builder, facilitator, and coordinator for the committee. He or she also serves as the liaison for the committee to the administration of the sponsoring institution.

- **Vice chair:** The vice chair supports the chair in all of his or her functions when the chair is unable to attend meetings or perform his or her duties. The vice chair may assist in resolving grievances during committee meetings. He or she may serve as the public face for the GMEC in the absence of the GMEC chair.

- **Nonvoting members:** Nonvoting members are appointed regular members or persons invited on an ad hoc basis for communication and input, but are not allowed to vote. Nonvoting members are usually asked to depart in closed sessions or when critical confidential information is being discussed. Examples of helpful nonvoting members include the president of the medical staff, chief medical officer, chief financial officer, additional house staff representatives, and GME program coordinators.

- **DIO:** The DIO ensures that the committee maintains compliance with ACGME or accrediting agency standards. The DIO must sign any program curricula changes that program directors make to programs before they are presented to the ACGME. Additional roles of the DIO include scheduling the internal review, selecting internal review subcommittees, and overseeing program applications and modifications.

- **Administrative member(s):** Administrative members serve as links between the administration and the medical education committee. They may present institutional changes and concerns, and report new strategies, policies, and procedures within the institution. Additionally, members of the committee may present concerns or inquiries to the administrative representatives to communicate back to the larger body. The administrative representatives may serve as advocates for the committee among executive leaders.

- **Program director(s):** Program directors are responsible for communicating important changes discussed in the GMEC to faculty and residents. The program director appointed to the GMEC must commit to regular attendance and participation in the GMEC and its function. He or she reports changes in program schedules, resident numbers, department guidelines, curricula, and evaluations, as well as any concerns or suggestions that relate to GME. Each program director may be asked to participate periodically in an internal review.

- **Resident representative(s):** The resident representatives of the GMEC are appointed by their peers to represent ideas and concerns of the graduate medical trainees within the institution. They must be committed to attending GMEC meetings. The duration of appointment is usually one year. At least one of the resident members should be a voting member.

- **Secretarial support:** The GMEC secretary keeps written minutes of all meetings and reports all motions and votes that occurred during the meetings. The secretary is responsible for maintaining all records of the GMEC, including new policies and guidelines, and ensuring that they are aligned with institutional policies. He or she is also responsible for collecting and maintaining minutes of all appointed GMEC subcommittees. These documents are important during the institutional review.

Developing a mission statement and goals

The ACGME requires that the sponsoring institution show evidence of its commitment to GME in a written document. One way to show your institution's commitment is by outlining it in a mission statement, created by the GMEC, DIO, administration, and other medical staff members, as well as medical education leaders. A mission statement serves to direct purpose, build collaborative effort, establish priorities and values, and align actions with goals and perspectives. The mission statement should be developed in conjunction with the overall mission of the ACGME, the sponsoring institution, academic leaders, and supporting partners.

The mission statement should:

- Be easily translated into action with available resources

- Clearly identify the organization's uniqueness

- Be targeted toward a specific audience

The overall goal of a mission statement is an end product that exemplifies excellence and quality in its commitment to GME. Goals outlined in the mission statement should be developed in collaborative efforts by administration, training programs, and those responsible for financing education and supporting staff. The goals must be tangible and obtainable.

Outlining the function of the GMEC in your institution

An institution's GMEC is vital in implementing the mission statement or joint commitment and monitoring the compliance of GME programs. The GMEC works collaboratively with both administration and the academic faculty and staff to carry out the institution's and committee's medical education mission and to give advice on all issues relating to GME. The GMEC is responsible for developing policies and guidelines that meet ACGME recommendations and requirements. It is also responsible for resident policies and guidelines specific to the sponsoring institution aligning with institutional policies and bylaws. (See the nine steps to successful guidelines and policies in Figure 1.2.)

FIGURE 1.2

Nine Steps to Successful Guidelines and Policies

Step 1: Discern between mandatory organizational policies, policies mandated by governing bodies, and policies and guidelines necessary for organize function of GME and GMEC.

Step 2: Understand the goals and reasoning for creating a new policy or guideline.

Step 3: Know your target audience.

Step 4: Discuss what is required to maintain compliance.

Step 5: Discuss the benefits and risk of noncompliance.

Step 6: Identify the people on your team or within your institution that are vital to the implementation of the policy.

Step 7: Brainstorm how to measure compliance.

Step 8: Evaluate outcomes once implemented.

Step 9: One year after implementation, revise policies and guidelines to meet unexpected needs that relate to the overall goals of the policy or guideline.

Specific responsibilities of the GMEC include:

- **Deliver an annual report to the sponsoring institution to review its financial commitment to the GME programs.** This includes resident cost, faculty cost, benefit packages, and additional funding for new resident positions or faculty. If your institution is not familiar with resident salary cost and needed benefits, this report might include a regional market analysis of salaries and benefits for residents and fellows in similar programs with similar responsibilities. (See Figure 1.3 for questions to consider regarding resident salaries and benefits.)

FIGURE 1.3

Questions to consider regarding salary and benefits for residents

1. What are the responsibilities of your residents and fellows?

2. Is the salary and benefits package competitive with those of other institutions in the market that might recruit the same applicants?

3. What is the right mix of direct pay and benefits that would communicate your commitment to quality medical education and recruitment?

4. What are standard benefits for residents in your region?

5. If the hospital hires residents, which benefits received by regular employees should you negotiate for residents?

6. Define the desired work culture or investigate the work culture of the sponsoring institution. Does the pay structure reflect the culture you desire? (Paying below the market may not result in a lower-quality applicant, and paying much higher might draw suspicion that the organization is desperate to recruit.)

Present answers to these questions to the administration along with supporting documentation of market salaries and benefits.

Estimating faculty cost analysis might include using faculty-to-resident ratios and average salaries in your region for the specialty, and incorporating rotation schedules or faculty time commitments for teaching.

- **Communicate with the medical staff committee to discuss patient safety and quality of care in resident education.** This communication can take place in several ways, including reports at routine medical staff meetings, e-mail messages, and an internal newsletter.

- **Promote communication among the institution, program directors, house staff, and administration.** Create opportunities for representatives from each group to participate on committees or activities related to improving GME or the work environment. The subcommittees can report back to the GMEC on their progress and findings.

- **Oversee communication between program directors and residents' rotation sites.** Program directors must communicate with the responsible faculty at institutions where residents rotate. The program director has the ultimate responsibility for the residents' education, compliance, and performance at the rotating site. The GMEC must monitor the communication between the program director and the participating institution.

- **Conduct internal reviews of training programs within the institution to ensure that they meet the standards of the accrediting agency.** The GMEC and DIO are responsible for conducting internal reviews and making recommendations to programs regarding citations, corrective actions, and any concerns reported from the internal review committee.

- **Review affiliation sites and programs to ensure compliance with accreditation agencies.** The sponsoring institution must verify that participating institutions and programs are accredited, adhering to ACGME guidelines, and have adequate resources to deliver quality resident education and oversee residents rotating in their institution. The sponsoring institution must ensure academic partners commit to resident supervison and duty hour guidelines.

- **Oversee institutional compliance with ACGME standards and requirements.** The GMEC must have governance over programs and resident responsibilities and duties. The GMEC is a good forum to review policies, new guidelines, agreements, and changes in curricula.

- **Review ACGME report letters and citations, and monitor programs for plans and implementation.** After a review of letters and citations, the GMEC should recommend potential solutions and corrective actions.

- **Develop policies and guidelines that ensure the quality of programs and a safe environment for patients and residents.** See Figure 1.4 for specific guidelines and policies the committee should develop.

FIGURE 1.4

GMEC roles in policy development and oversight

Policies the ACGME requires the GMEC to develop and oversee	Examples of policies the GMEC may help the institution to develop	GME program policies the ACGME requires the GMEC to oversee
Resident duty hours	Medical records completion	Resident recruitment, selection, and promotion
Resident supervision	Resident and student rotators observation	Leave of absence and program extension
Resident selections, appointments, and dismissals	External rotators impact	Program resident supervision
Curricula oversight and evaluation	Mandatory compliance testing	Moonlighting
Leave of absence	Recruitment	Duty hours
Grievance and due process	Internet and e-mail	
Moonlighting	Expansion of residency programs	
Physician impairment	Implementing new residency training	
Harassment	Implementing program changes	
Accommodation for disabilities	Vendor interactions	
GME program closures and reductions		
Disaster response		

Additional functions of the GMEC may be specific to the local organization. In institutions with nonaccredited programs or programs from several accrediting agencies, the GMEC may be charged to monitor programs to ensure that they meet equivalent standards that satisfy all accrediting agencies.

The DIO

The DIO has a major role in the oversight of program compliance and administration of the ACGME programs.[1] The institution must establish guidelines for selecting, appointing, and hiring a skilled DIO. The institution's accreditation rests on the DIO's ability to combine education, quality, professionalism, and technical skills while overseeing the training programs within the institution.

The ACGME mandates that each sponsoring institution appoint a DIO to carry out the following responsibilities within the institution:

- **Review and sign any documents submitted to the ACGME regarding program changes or citations that would have a major impact on the program or sponsoring institution.** Examples of these documents and changes include expansion of residency programs, implementation of innovative programs that are not standard to ACGME guidelines, responses to program citations, the addition of trainees that might impinge upon GME training and resources, and program changes in leadership.

- **Establish a designee to sign documents in the DIO's absence.** This is important to ensure that the GME office continues to function when the DIO must be away.

- **Assist the GMEC chair in presenting the annual report to the sponsoring institution, if necessary.** The DIO is vital to reporting duty hours, program changes, institutional responses to citations, and updates regarding ACGME changes and requirements.

- **Review program complaints before they are sent to the ACGME.** The DIO is the institutional representative responsible for reporting any resident complaints to the ACGME. The program director or designee is responsible for listening to and evaluating complaints within the specific program.

- **Improve GME through program development and implementation.** The DIO must work to continually improve the resident learning environment by collaborating with leaders in the sponsoring institution and overseeing the structure of the GMEC and GME programs.

- **Support the institution's program directors.** The DIO supports the program directors by assisting with the completion of program information forms for the ACGME, recommending responses to ACGME site visit findings and citations, providing leadership training, and ensuring a safe workplace environment for residents. The DIO is responsible for working with the GMEC to coordinate policy and guideline development, assess safety in the work setting, and plan for unexpected adverse events such as natural disasters, institutional closures, and other emergencies.

HOW THE INSTITUTIONAL REVIEW AFFECTS THE PROGRAM REVIEW AND VICE VERSA

The success of the institutional review is important to the maintenance of all GME programs within the sponsoring institution. If the institution is not accredited, GME programs will also lose accreditation. If multiple programs are not accredited, the ACGME may see that as unfavorable during an institutional site visit. The GMEC and DIO must clearly identify areas of need and communicate this with program directors at each GMEC meeting, during internal reviews, and through ongoing communication. Both GMEC and non-GMEC members must be educated on the teamwork needed to accomplish a favorable report from the ACGME during institutional and program site visits.

The institutional review and the program review require the commitment of the sponsoring institution, participating sites, other program directors, the teaching staff, the hospital leaders and staff, and residents. The overall goal of the surveyors is to assess the quality of education and compliance with ACGME requirements.

Common responsibilities of the sponsoring institution and the GME programs include:

- Establishing and maintaining program requirements at the sponsoring institution and participating sites

- Identifying and supplying appropriate resources, space, time, and finances to meet the educational mission of the institution and the program and to meet the requirements of the governing bodies

- Ensuring that program and institutional affiliation agreements are up to date

- Developing and implementing policies for resident selection, appointment, and approval

- Establishing policies and procedures to ensure resident well-being and patient safety

- Developing a high-quality educational program that meets ACGME standards

TRAINING NON-GMEC MEMBERS ON THE INSTITUTIONAL REVIEW

Administrators and employees may not be familiar with GME oversight and may have limited knowledge of the ACGME and/or its requirements. The medical education leadership, GMEC, and DIO are responsible for educating their partners about the organization of medical education, the accrediting agency, and the importance of compliance to policies and requirements. Suspected barriers to training non-GMEC members are time constraints for administrators and employees, a lack of well-defined communications, a limited forum to present information to non-GMEC members, and limited knowledge of others about their role in the accreditation process.

Developing a process for delivering education related to the GMEC must begin with the GMEC and DIO. The following are the steps they should take:

1. Discuss the importance of collaboration with the administration and sponsoring institution to develop the best model to address and respond to GME matters.

2. Review the ACGME institutional requirements (IRs), common program requirements, and program specialty-specific requirements.

3. Consider appointing GMEC members to report on certain aspects of the IRs and their program-specific requirements at subsequent GMEC meetings and at the next program department meeting or medical staff meeting.

4. Ask administrators, educators, GMEC members, faculty, and residents for suggestions on how to make this effort effective.

5. Ask the GMEC and subcommittee members to suggest methods of communication and formats for presentation.

6. Poll the GMEC members to see what other committees are represented among the group.

7. Appoint committee members to discuss GMEC and IRs as they relate to the other committee's goal.

8. Present findings to both the GMEC and institution committees.

The GMEC and the DIO should also discuss alternative methods to deliver important information regarding IRs and the institutional review (e.g., institutional newsletters, departmental newsletters, meeting announcements, training courses, and e-mail). The brief communications and trainings should include reviewing the institutional review instructions and IRD, discussing appropriate responses to the questions asked on the IRD, explaining the importance of the institutional review, and providing information that is helpful in completing the IRD.

COMMUNICATING THE INSTITUTIONAL REVIEW TO THE PROGRAM DIRECTORS AND CHAIRS

Program directors and chairs must be educated on the IRs and the role of the sponsoring institution. Program directors can receive information during GMEC and subcommittee meetings. However, the sponsoring institution and primary department must also invest money and resources to develop qualified leaders for medical education to sustain a viable training program. Directors and leaders need to attend and become actively involved in multiple academic organizations or attend multiple training programs.

To deliver information about the institutional review within the institution, GMEC members can do some or all of the following:

- Give a 20-minute session on the institutional review at a medical staff meeting

- Give a short presentation to the administration

- Have a roundtable session with office administrative staff on how to assist program directors and chairs

- Give grand rounds on medical education and site visits

- Present a mini-workshop on the process

COLLABORATION IS KEY IN PLANNING FOR REVIEWS

Changes and expectations in medicine and GME are sometimes met with apprehension from administration, faculty, trainees, and support staff. The ability to navigate through requirements is paramount to success.

Here are some steps for the DIO that are helpful in the navigation process:

- Choose the lead person who will be responsible for assisting the DIO with the project outcome.

- Consider creating small committees to organize a systematic approach to preparing for the review. Include members from administration (e.g., key executives that are responsible for GME support), program directors, and academic leaders from the institution's GME office, resident representatives, and the DIO.

- Delegate a member of the GMEC to lead a systems review of the institution's GME status. Then, have the member review those findings with the DIO before submitting them to the full GMEC.

- Review the IRs, the IRD, and common program requirements. Look for similar sections that all parties can work toward.

- Review comments and responses on the IRD to ensure that they reflect the current state of the institution and that they address every aspect of the ACGME requirements.

- Highlight inherent risk areas to address before IRD submission.

- Establish a timeline to report and communicate with the DIO.

- Create an institutional checklist with tasks to be performed, the date recognized, associated documentation, the name of the person(s) responsible for the task, potential risk areas, suggestions for resolution, and a completion date. (See the example of an institutional checklist in Figure 1.5.)

- Set a date for the final assessment before submitting the documents.

- Set a date to review submitted information before the site visit.

- Check schedules well in advance to ensure that key members of GME and administration are available to do an assessment before the site review.

Further discussion of these steps will be included in a later chapter. The next chapter will provide an overview of the institutional organization and responsibilities.

FIGURE 1.5

Institutional Checklist

☐ Review Institutional requirements, institutional review document, common program requirements, and program-specific requirements for specialty

☐ Check accreditation of sponsoring institution and participating institutions

☐ Secure written commitment statement of sponsoring institution

☐ Identify key GME leaders

☐ Identify designee to sign important documents that must be submitted to ACGME in absence of DIO

☐ Verify institutional support to GME (i.e., financial, resources, space, technology etc.)

☐ Verify protected time of DIO, program directors and key GME leadership

☐ Review resident rotation schedules

☐ Confirm Program Letters of Agreements for rotations

☐ Confirm Master Affiliation agreements for major participating sites

☐ Review and update required written policies (See Fig. 1.4)

☐ Verify financial support for residents

☐ Check Agreement of Appointment for required components

☐ Check current professional liability policy of residents for required components

☐ Get Duty Hour reports from programs

☐ Check availability of resident counseling services

☐ Review availability of resident confidential reporting for concerns and exchange of information

☐ Check adequacy of ancillary support services

FIGURE 1.5

❑ Check availability of resident food services, call rooms, and safety

❑ Review GMEC composition, function, and reporting lines

❑ Verify adequate communication between GMEC, institution, medical staff, and program director

❑ Check annual report for required elements and appropriate reporting

❑ Verify internal review occurred midway between last accreditation visit and next site visit

❑ Check internal review report for ACGME required elements

ENDNOTES

1. Risenberg, L.A., Rosenbaum, P.F., and Stick, S.L. 2006. "Competencies, Essential Training and Resources Viewed by Designated Institutional Officials as Important to the Position in Graduate Medical Education." *Academic Medicine* 81 (5): 431.

INSTITUTIONAL ORGANIZATION AND RESPONSIBILITIES

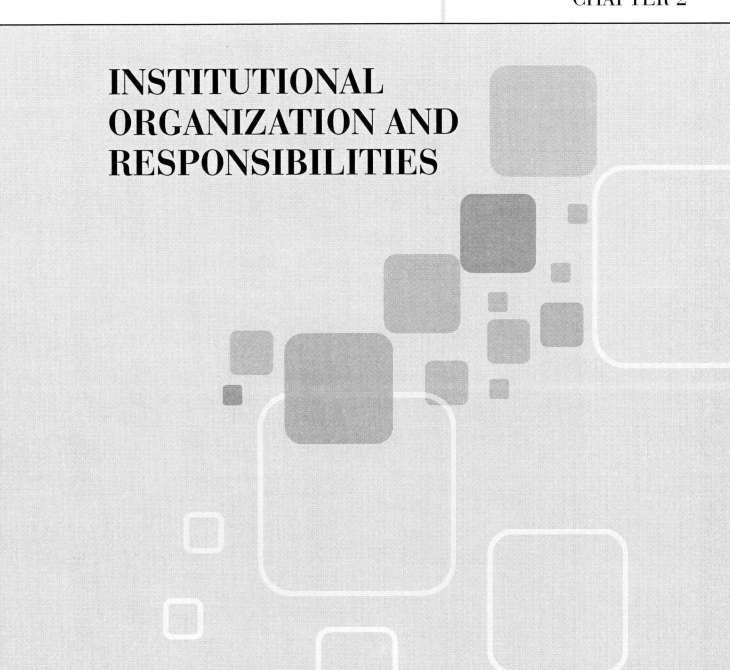

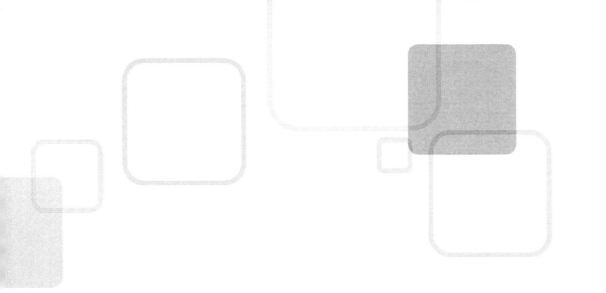

INSTITUTIONAL ORGANIZATION AND RESPONSIBILITIES

When the Accreditation Council for Graduate Medical Education (ACGME) comes to your organization for the institutional review, its site visitors will expect to see that everyone in the institution has an appropriate understanding of the graduate medical education (GME) program. It's the sponsoring institution's responsibility to clearly educate all staff members and leaders about the organization's commitment to GME.

Those involved in GME—the designated institutional official (DIO), graduate medical education committee (GMEC) members, other GME leaders, and residents—must also understand the sponsoring institution's organizational structure.

During the institutional review, the ACGME site visitor may interview any of these individuals to verify their support and commitment to GME. Each person must understand his or her role and the role of the key leaders in the institution. The ACGME's objective is to verify previously reported information in GME documents, residents' surveys, and GME policies.

The sponsoring institution must have an organizational structure that the staff, GMEC members, residents, and other employees can easily identify and recognize. Most institutions demonstrate their leadership rank and structure

---

in an organizational chart. The organizational chart must show the rank of the administrative system that oversees the GME programs in the sponsoring institution. (See Figure 2.1 for an example of an organizational chart.)

An understanding of the sponsoring institution's organizational structure is also important to ensure that the mission and goals of GME and the institution are aligned, to understand the source of funding, and to enhance collaborative efforts that will improve the longevity of medical education within the institution.

When preparing for the institutional review, it is important to review the following with the institutional administration and staff, GMEC members and GME leaders, faculty, residents, and other staff members who might be potential interviewees for the institutional review:

- The history of the sponsoring institution with regard to medical education

- The organizational structure

- Medical school linkages

- The purpose and function of the sponsoring institution in any educational consortium membership, if applicable

- Changes in leadership since the last ACGME site visit

- Changes in governance since the last ACGME site visit

- Changes in affiliations since the last ACGME site visit

- Actions taken to address previous citations from institutional reviews or program-specific citations noted on program reviews

The sponsoring institution must understand its role in electing and appointing the appropriate personnel to assist in carrying out responsibilities and changes necessary to meet requirements for ACGME accreditation.

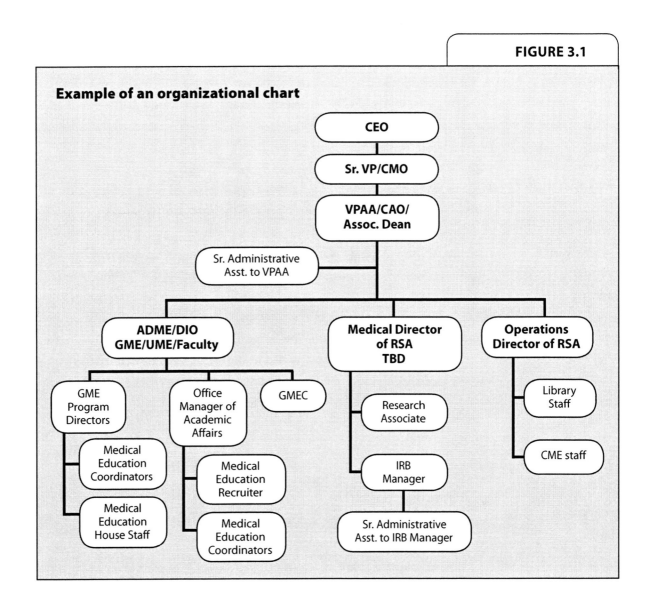

FIGURE 3.1

Example of an organizational chart

IDENTIFYING ORGANIZATIONAL RESOURCES FOR EDUCATION

The sponsoring institution must commit to providing adequate resources for GME, quality education, and quality patient care. The sponsoring institution must also commit to representation on the GMEC or a process to exchange information regarding major institutional initiations and changes that might affect GME.

The DIO and GMEC must be familiar with lead contact persons in the institution, who are instrumental in helping to acquire needed personnel, space, facilities, technology, and learning resources, as well as securing affiliation or program agreements for outside rotations. The DIO and GME leadership must also be knowledgeable about the institution's budget cycle and fiscal goals.

The financial support of the GME programs requires committed leadership in both the institution and the GME department. The DIO and/or designated GME leaders must have a clear understanding of how funds are allocated for medical education and how to get funding to support changes in GME programs, resource needs, education, and personnel growth. The DIO and GMEC must communicate openly with the sponsoring institution regarding concerns, achievements, needed growth, and potential adverse reports.

The DIO, GMEC, and GME leadership can begin to identify organizational resources by communicating with their immediate supervisors. The supervisors are the first line for identifying the administrative leaders that are key to providing support staff, additional funding, new facilities, restructuring of old facilities, technology, legal advice, learning tools, support for a larger budget for GME, and so on. Institution directories, institutional organization charts, and committee rosters may also be helpful in identifying persons that are vital to the success of GME within the institution. For example, identifying the director of pharmacy and discussing with him or her resident practice in writing and filling prescriptions may be helpful in reducing pharmacy errors in the institution. Another example is to identify the IT director and get his or her help to develop a method to capture duty hours through payroll and the resident management system. (See Figure 2.2 for examples of institutional teamwork in addressing GME needs.)

FIGURE 2.2

Examples of institutional teamwork in addressing GME needs

Need	Institutional team	Resource or contribution
New computers within GME programs	IT department including chief information officer and director, chief financial officer or designee, chief operating officer or planning operations, administrative representative, GME representative	Assist with planning for purchase, develop budget, and develop business proposal including allocation of computers, purchasing, space negotiation, implementation of network systems, and software choice expertise
Reduce pharmacy errors among residents and staff	Pharmacy staff and director, IT support, GME representative, nursing representative, resident representative	Group planning to review data and report prior to initiation of change, developing new process to decrease errors, planning for evaluation and reporting of information after project initiation, and measuring impact of decreased errors within the institution
Resident supervision	Quality committee, DIO, GMEC, program directors, residents, CMO, medical staff, nursing staff, GME leaders	Review quality of patient care as it relates to resident supervision, and engagement of nursing staff, faculty, residents, other hospital staff members, and the quality committee in monitoring and reporting

THE SPONSORING INSTITUTION'S RESPONSIBILITIES

The sponsoring institution must commit to providing resources and support to promote professionalism, ethical behavior, and personal development of residents. An institution that does not comply with ACGME guidelines and recommendations risks losing accreditation for all of its GME programs. In its institutional requirements (IRs), the ACGME states that the sponsoring institution—including the governance, administration, and GME leadership—must do the following:

- Review, date, and sign a document that outlines the institution's commitment to GME within at least one year prior to the institutional review

- Commit to ensuring compliance with the ACGME IRs, common program requirements (CPRs), and program-specific requirements

- Commit to safe patient care through adequate resident supervision, quality curricula and education, strong interpersonal and communication skills, system-based learning, and frequent evaluation and assessment of resident competency

- Appoint a program director for each GME program

- Appoint key leaders within the organization to champion the implementation of its mission statement and to ensure that GME programs meet ACGME requirements

- Ensure that agreements with participating institutions are not expired or more than five years old

- Monitor participating institutions for compliance with ACGME guidelines

- Promote professional, ethical behavior and personal development of residents

- Provide DIO and program directors with sufficient resources, finances, and time to effectively carry out their responsibilities

Professional behavior and personal development of residents

Promoting professional, ethical behavior and personal development in residents requires a collaborative approach that involves the support of the sponsoring institution, GMEC, and medical staff, as well as the creativity of the GME office and program directors, and the cooperation of residents. Developing activities to foster *professionalism* in both residents and the teaching staff must include a conscious effort to maintain quality, respect for others, trustworthiness, competence, and integrity. Maintaining professional behavior within the environment requires the ability to monitor and report behavior and activity that is not professional in a supportive manner with modeling of appropriate behavior to achieve competent qualified physicians.

Examples of activities for residents and program directors, which can be jointly sponsored or led by the sponsoring institution and the GME program, to meet these requirements include:

- Customer service training

- Promoting community volunteerism

- Encouraging resident participation in multicultural events to promote communication with diverse populations

- Developing programs to teach the importance of confidentiality of patient information

- Organizing team events to develop quality programs that focus on delivering the highest standard of care (e.g., models of care for the most common illnesses within the institution; best examples for delivering high-quality customer service; team efforts to study and implement programs to improve employee morale, communication, and satisfaction)

- Modeling of high standards and integrity by institutional leaders and GME leaders

Development of *ethical behavior* is not as straightforward. Although no distinct activities are confirmed as sure ways to teach ethical behavior, the sponsoring institution and GME programs can promote ethics in the following ways:

- Outlining in writing specific guidelines for ethical behavior

- Establishing consequences in writing for noncompliance with ethical behavior guidelines

- Promoting trust among employees, residents, faculty, and the staff

- Being careful to avoid micromanagement

- Offering appreciation and awards to residents who display strong ethical behavior and provide examples of accountability

Personal development is important to producing a well-rounded quality physician. Residents will naturally progress during training with either a positive or a negative attitude toward training and medicine based on their personal or shared experiences during the training period. The sponsoring institution and GME leaders must commit to fostering an environment that promotes quality and effective learning, self-motivation, and open exchange of information between residents and staff members. The institution must include residents in some of the decision-making activities related to their training. This will enforce the importance of their participation and impact on the overall experience in education and patient care, improve the strength of the relationship between the GME departments and residents, improve the institution's awareness of resident impact, and help to frame personal values as it relates to quality patient care and human interactions.

If communication and teamwork are avoided, the resident may experience imbalance, intellectual and physical overload, and stagnant personal growth. The sponsoring institution, program directors, and residents must all understand the need for balance with commitment to ongoing learning and personal development.

Examples of activities that are used in GME programs to improve resident personal development are:

- Resident support groups

- Peer tutoring and mentoring

- Seminars from personal development coaches

- Presentations from local and regional leaders

- Faculty mentors and coaches for residents

Regardless of the planned activity, the GME office and sponsoring institution must be supportive to residents and program directors and be willing to explore opportunities that enhance achievement, self-motivation, institutional participation, and perpetual self-learning by residents.

THE INSTITUTION'S GME POLICIES AND PROCEDURES

The sponsoring institution must develop GME policies and procedures that provide guidance in maintaining quality education, enhancing resident and patient safety, and ensuring the ongoing accreditation for both the sponsoring institution and the training program. In addition, these policies and procedures must clearly outline the organization's procedures for handling matters related to GME and residents.

Examples of newer or changing ACGME requirements include a:

- Resident supervision policy

- Disruptive resident behavior policy

- Duty hours policy

Each policy addresses three major ACGME goals for resident training: resident education, patient safety, and professionalism.

Resident supervision policy
The resident supervision policy for all programs must require that qualified faculty supervise residents in clinical areas to promote continued education and quality care for patients.

Program-specific supervision policies are also necessary to ensure that residents have optimal learning environments, maintain patient safety, and maintain resident safety while experiencing fatigue. The institutional supervision policy sets guidelines for monitoring residents and providing oversight for quality education while at the sponsoring institution and all participating facilities.

The sponsoring institution must be prepared to support GME leaders in implementing the policy. The sponsoring institution and DIO must be fully aware of the supervision policy in sites where residents rotate. This policy must be included in program agreements with an understanding that the sponsoring institution's policy does not supersede the policies of the participating rotation site.

For example, in the sponsoring institution residents may be allowed to function with some autonomy as they progress in their postgraduate levels, but in the participating institution, residents may not be allowed to function unsupervised at any level.

Documents that are helpful in creating the supervision policy include:

- ACGME institutional requirements

- ACGME common program requirements (CPRs)

- ACGME program-specific requirements

- Centers for Medicare & Medicaid Services guidelines regarding resident supervision

- The sponsoring institution's policies and guidelines

- Participating institutions' policies and guidelines

- The Joint Commission standards for resident supervision

The sponsoring institution must maintain accreditation with The Joint Commission and ACGME. A well-written policy takes into consideration requirements and recommendations from all governing bodies, local institutional policies, and policies of participating rotation sites.

The sponsoring institution's policy on resident supervision must contain:

- Roles and responsibilities of administrative leaders of the sponsoring institution, GME leaders, the DIO, residents and fellows, program directors, and program coordinators in implementing the policy

- Role of the supervising faculty

- Procedures for monitoring resident supervision

- Personnel responsible for monitoring resident supervision

- Procedures to evaluate results of monitoring and to implement a feedback mechanism that would improve quality of care and supervision

Program resident supervision policies must contain:

- Roles and responsibilities of residents and fellows, program directors, and program coordinators

- Description of residents' graduated levels of experience

- Role of upper-level residents and interns

- Role of the supervising faculty

- Procedures for monitoring resident supervision

- Procedures for evaluating residents and addressing issues that affect patient care, resident learning experiences, and resident safety

Disruptive resident behavior policy

Disruptive behavior can interfere with training activities, patient care, resident learning, instruction, and professional growth. Establishing clear guidelines and procedures for dealing with the disruptive resident, faculty member, or staff member is important to optimizing the learning environment and promoting a safe workplace. The sponsoring institution must clearly define disruptive behavior, the consequences for it, and how the consequences will be enforced.

The disruptive resident behavior policy must address:

- Sexual harassment

- Abusive language or actions toward patients, residents, faculty, or the staff

- Injury to person or property

- Loud noises

- Lack of cooperation of residents with other peers and staff members

- Racial or ethnic comments

- Any act that interferes with the normal activities of employment and patient care

- Procedures for reporting disruptive behavior, including confidential reporting, if applicable

- Procedures for addressing the disruptive behavior

- Guidelines for appeal and a fair hearing process

- Guidelines for probation

- Guidelines for dismissal

Duty hours policy

For many years, residents and fellows worked long hours providing care for patients, completing administrative duties related to patient care, and performing overnight duties. The ACGME now requires that the sponsoring institution have written policies to address resident duty hours. In 2003, the ACGME approved standards that decreased resident work hours to improve patient safety and risk of harm to residents related to fatigue. The duty hours policy must be implemented in every sponsoring institution and GME program. The sponsoring institution must work in collaboration with the DIO to develop a policy that meets ACGME requirements.

The sponsoring institution is responsible for developing the following:

- A written duty hours policy that is highly visible to the institution, the GMEC, GME leaders, hospital staff, and residency programs

- A procedure to monitor duty hours

The ACGME has set the following guidelines to define duty hour restrictions:

- Residents must not work more than 80 hours weekly over an average of four weeks

- Residents must receive one day off weekly averaged over four weeks

- Residents must be given adequate time for rest

- Residents must not work more than 30 hours in any given assignment

- Residents cannot accept new patients after a 24-hour period of work

Managing duty hours can be an arduous task for program directors and residents. Many electronic systems are available to assist in this responsibility. These systems can record resident schedules, internal moonlighting, didactic conferences, and nonclinical hours.

The GMEC and DIO will assist by:

- Delegating specific assignments to program directors in logging duty hours

- Training program coordinators in the use of the logging system

- Setting deadlines for receiving duty hour reports from program directors

- Verifying the recording of duty hours

- Developing an action plan to address noncompliance to duty hours logging, reporting, and adherence requirements

- Developing a mechanism to evaluate corrective action for previous noncompliance with duty hours requirements

INSTITUTIONAL RESPONSIBILITIES FOR RESIDENTS

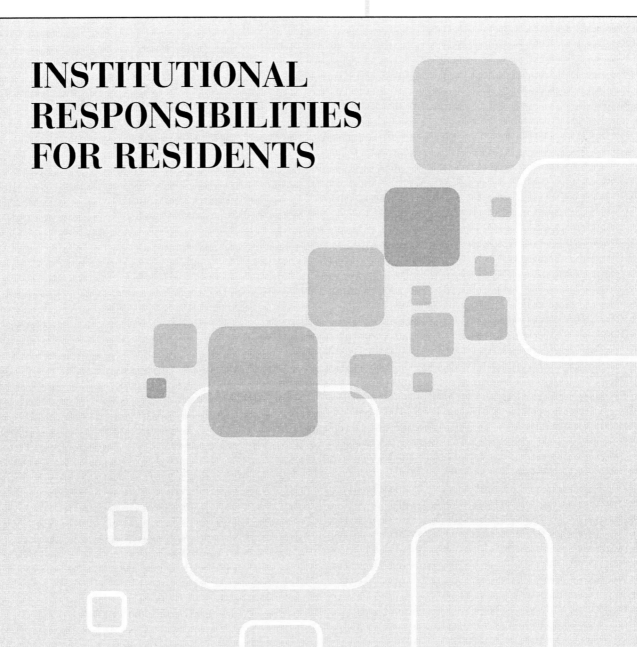

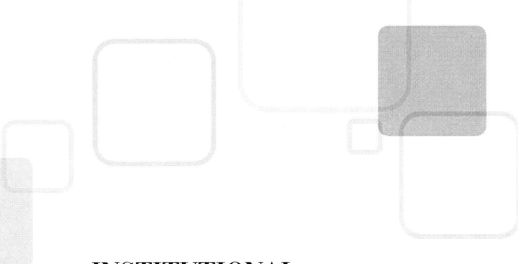

INSTITUTIONAL RESPONSIBILITIES FOR RESIDENTS

The sponsoring institution must develop policies to address resident selection, approval, and appointment for training. The resident hiring process has become a complex issue involving human resources, compliance standards set by hospital governing bodies, and workforce laws. The sponsoring institution must also meet the Accreditation Council for Graduate Medical Education (ACGME) requirements and The Joint Commission accreditation standards for the hospital. The goal of these requirements is to ensure patient safety by hiring a quality medical staff.

The ACGME will request verification that the sponsoring institution and graduate medical education committee (GMEC) has written policies for selecting and appointing residents. According to the ACGME institutional requirements (IRs), sponsoring institutions must assess the eligibility of applicants. To be eligible, applicants must have graduated from medical school. If they graduated from a medical school outside the United States or Canada, they must have one of the following:

- A currently valid certificate from the Educational Commission for Foreign Medical Graduates.

- A full, unrestricted license to practice medicine where they are training.

- Proof of completion of a "Fifth Pathway" program provided by a medical school accredited by the Liaison Committee on Medical Education. A Fifth Pathway program is an academic year of supervised clinical education for foreign students who meet certain criteria.

The selection process for residents must be a nondiscriminatory process in which residents are selected or excluded based on program-related criteria. Selection and appointment criteria must be careful to adhere to written institutional policies regarding hiring and reviewing applicants with disabilities. The ACGME urges each institution to have a policy regarding the hiring of disabled applicants. The ACGME highly recommends that, when possible, sponsoring institutions use an organized matching program such as the national resident matching program to find qualified resident candidates.

As part of its resident interviewing and hiring process, the sponsoring institution must:

- Ensure that only eligible applicants are selected

- Ensure that applicants have the appropriate credentials

- Provide applicants with current information about program benefits, liability coverage, and resources at the institution

- Ensure that hiring practices are nondiscriminatory

- Provide each resident with a written agreement of appointment

- Make a commitment to provide a safe and fair work environment

- Provide residents with written policies for grievances and due process

- Provide a statement of liability coverage, including the amount of coverage, items covered, and exclusions

DEVELOPING APPROPRIATE CRITERIA FOR SELECTION OF RESIDENTS

The IRs give clear instructions on eligibility for entrance into a residency program. However, the sponsoring institution may have additional screening guidelines that must be performed prior to hire, including:

- Background checks, including Office of Inspector General screening for Medicare and Medicaid sanctions

- Drug screens

- State medical board rehabilitation requirements

- Medical screenings

The designated institutional official (DIO) must work closely with the sponsoring institution to ensure that a resident meets all eligibility requirements for both ACGME and the sponsoring institution before signing the resident agreement.

DEVELOPING APPROPRIATE CRITERIA FOR EVALUATION, PROMOTION, AND TERMINATION OF RESIDENTS

Each program director must develop guidelines for evaluation and promotion of residents to the next postgraduate level. These criteria are based on standards set by the ACGME and the program-specific residency review committees. Residents not meeting these criteria are subject to probation, suspension, and dismissal. The institution must have in place a written policy to address criteria for probation, suspension, and dismissal.

Examples of areas of performance that may warrant probation, suspension, and termination include:

- **Professional performance:** Actions that endanger patients or the staff, violations of institutional policies, and actions which are detrimental to the institution and program

- **Academic performance:** Actions that display knowledge deficits, including the inability to perform assignments in a manner commensurate with postgraduate-level education and the inability to apply learned skills in an appropriate manner

Residents with professional or academic performance issues which warrant review may be given several options, including:

- Performance improvement plan

- Probation

- Temporary suspension

- Termination from the program and institution

The ACGME requires the sponsoring institution to give a resident at least a four-month written notice when his or her performance is unfavorable for promotion or the program is considering termination. The sponsoring institution, GMEC, and all graduate medical education (GME) programs must have written policies that outline the procedures for nonpromotion or dismissal. The DIO, GMEC, and program directors may find it necessary to seek legal counsel in some nonpromotion and dismissal cases. The initial agreement for hire must spell out the duration of the appointment and a statement for renewal, which specifies that reappointments occur on the basis of evaluation and successful completion of all requirements for the contracted period. The initial agreement must inform the resident that the institution has a process for grievance and fair hearing in circumstances where promotion and termination are a concern.

The sponsoring institution must have a written outlined process for handling educational performance issues, noncompliance with institutional policies, and issues related to patient safety concerns. When reviewing evaluation and reasons for nonrenewal of appointments, the resident must be allowed a fair hearing and due process, such as the one outlined in the flow chart in Figure 3.1.

The written fair hearing or grievance process must include the following components:

- Criteria for requesting a fair hearing, including who can request one and the appropriate time to request one

- What steps the institution will take when the fair hearing is requested

- What happens during the process

- How the results will be reported

- How long the process will take

- Who can be present during the fair hearing process

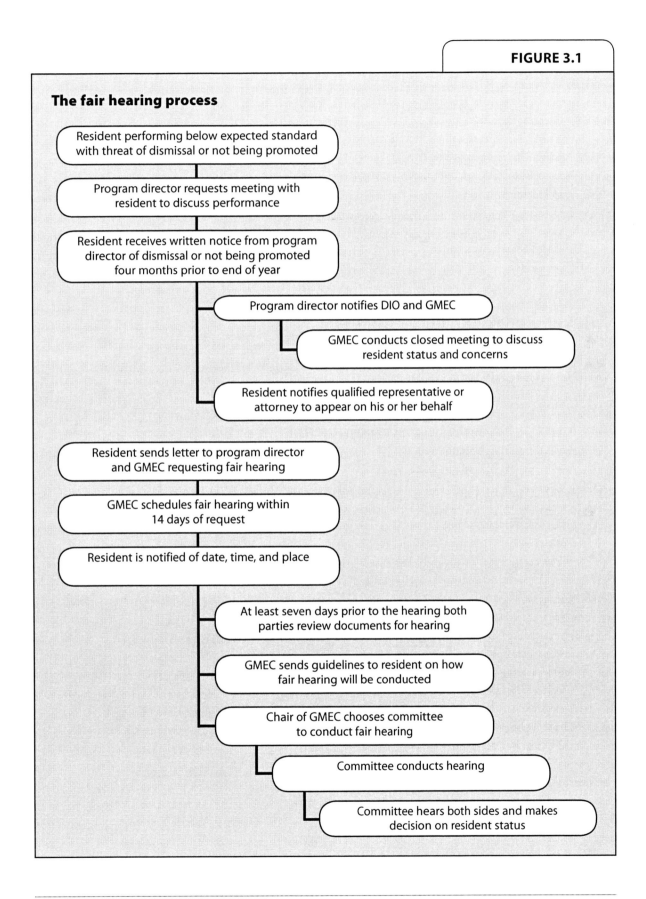

FIGURE 3.1

The fair hearing process

Resident performing below expected standard with threat of dismissal or not being promoted

Program director requests meeting with resident to discuss performance

Resident receives written notice from program director of dismissal or not being promoted four months prior to end of year

Program director notifies DIO and GMEC

GMEC conducts closed meeting to discuss resident status and concerns

Resident notifies qualified representative or attorney to appear on his or her behalf

Resident sends letter to program director and GMEC requesting fair hearing

GMEC schedules fair hearing within 14 days of request

Resident is notified of date, time, and place

At least seven days prior to the hearing both parties review documents for hearing

GMEC sends guidelines to resident on how fair hearing will be conducted

Chair of GMEC chooses committee to conduct fair hearing

Committee conducts hearing

Committee hears both sides and makes decision on resident status

- Who makes the final decision in the fair hearing process

- What the possible outcomes are in the fair hearing process (i.e., probation, suspension, termination, reappointment)

When a case is strictly related to academic issues, the institution may keep the fair hearing sessions closed to all except the GMEC-appointed committee, the program director, the involved resident, and a qualified representative to act on the resident's behalf. However, the GMEC and the institution might choose to include legal representation for both the resident and the institution when resident issues involve noncompliance with institutional policies, decisions interfere with resident career development, or issues relate to more than academic performance.

FINANCIAL SUPPORT FOR RESIDENTS

The GME leadership and GMEC must make annual recommendations to the institution regarding the salaries and benefits of residents. Financial support must be sufficient to cover reasonable resident living expenses. The human resources department can assist in providing cost-of-living information, recommended benefits, and compensation. Items routinely included in a resident compensation package include:

- Health and dental benefits for the resident and his or her family (with health insurance benefits beginning the first day of the program)

- Liability coverage

- Professional development funds

- Continuing medical education days

- Allowance for pagers, computers or pocket PCs, and/or phones

- Vacation time (three to four weeks, depending on the postgraduate year level)

- Leave for family care or medical care (required by the Family Medical Leave Act for qualified employees)

- Annuity plan

- Health club membership

- Travel reimbursement

- Relocation reimbursement

- Any other items offered to employees of the sponsoring institution

Residents should be reasonably compensated with finances and resources to allow maximum learning experiences.

AGREEMENT OF APPOINTMENT

The agreement of appointment is important to maintain good working relationships among the sponsoring institution, resident, and GME office. The institution, DIO, GME leadership, and a legal representative must review the written agreement. According to the IRs, the contents of the initial agreement must include:

- Expectations of the resident

- Duration of the appointment (most appointments are renewed annually)

- Terms for renewal

- Salary and benefits

- Insurance coverage (health, dental, and disability)

- Allowances

- Liability coverage type, amount, and explanations (coverage during training may not pertain to residents who are moonlighting)

Other attachments might include:

- Resident supervision policy

- Moonlighting policy, including additional requirements such as liability for moonlighting activities, Drug Enforcement Administration number, and National Provider Identifier number

- Requirements for hospital compliance training

- Duty hours policy

- Medical records policy

Institutions may alternatively place these items in a resident manual and request documentation or a signature attesting that the resident has received and/or read the materials as part of the formal appointment agreement.

The institution must ensure that residents have the opportunity to receive support for medical, psychological, and social challenges. The ACGME mandates that institutions have policies to address harassment, physician impairment, substance abuse, and provisions for treatment and counseling when warranted.

DISASTER POLICY

The sponsoring institution and GMEC must also develop a process for notifying residents of program reductions, closures, and loss of accreditation. The ACGME may at times declare a "disaster." A disaster is defined as any event that interrupts more than one residency training program in the sponsoring institution. The GMEC and DIO must make contact with the ACGME within 10 days of a disaster to develop an alternative plan for resident education.

The ACGME requires every institution to have a policy that addresses disaster planning, including, but not limited to, natural disasters, facility interruption in care, institutional closure, and program closures. The plan must detail how residents will be notified of the disaster within 30 days. The policy must address the institution's steps to notify residents and to assist residents with transfer to another available program. It must also address steps regarding resident compensation and period of commitment. The transfer may be temporary or permanent based on the type of disaster or cause of closure and the recommendation of the ACGME. The DIO of the sponsoring institution must work closely with the ACGME to restore programs.

RESIDENT PARTICIPATION IN EDUCATIONAL AND PROFESSIONAL ACTIVITIES

The sponsoring institution and GMEC must allow an opportunity for resident participation in planning and delivering educational activities. The ACGME also requires resident participation on institutional committees. The sponsoring institution determines appointees to committees and, thus, may determine whether resident participation is allowed on specific committees. For those committees that are allowed, the residents are chosen for the committees by peer selection. The participation in educational programs and committees must fulfill the requirements of teaching the ACGME competencies and be a learning experience for the residents. Examples of educational activities and committees that residents can participate in to demonstrate these requirements include:

- GMEC

- Institutional peer review committees

- Quality committees

- Curriculum committees

- Ethics committee

- Promotions committee

- Evaluations committee

- Institutional review boards

- Institution planning committees

- Pharmacy and therapeutics committee

- Strategic planning committee

- Morbidity and mortality conferences

- Multidisciplinary tumor boards

- Presentations at grand rounds conferences

- Institutional research days

- Journal club activities

- Training on physician impairment

RESIDENT EDUCATIONAL AND WORK ENVIRONMENT

Resident education and patient safety are the two major objectives of GME training. The sponsoring institution must ensure that resident education takes precedence over the institution's service needs. The institution must commit to adequate providers, support staff, resources for recording patient care visits, and support services. It must also provide residents with adequate work space, technology, and supplies, time to complete assignments, food provisions, and secure and safe work environments.

Many institutions have implemented programs to improve safety for residents, such as:

- Training workshops for self-protection

- Escort services for residents leaving the hospital after hours

- Links to local police services for enhanced security

- Specific phone lines to call in case of emergency

- Contingency plans for extreme situations, such as hostage situations, fire, bomb threats, and so on

CONFIDENTIAL REPORTING FOR RESIDENTS

In most institutions, employees have a confidential way to report concerns to administration and institutional leaders about recurring problems or misconduct. Residents must be given the same opportunity. The sponsoring institution must work with the GMEC to develop a reporting mechanism that is nonpunitive and allows for fair and confidential reporting. Residents must have an opportunity to report issues related to both the educational and work environments.

The policy on reporting concerns regarding misconduct in the educational and work environments should describe:

- What the institution will do to make sure all residents know that such a process exists

- Where and to whom residents should report concerns

- A guarantee of confidentiality and protection for the person reporting

- Steps the administration should take when the report is received

- Who will respond and set corrective actions to concerns

- When it is appropriate to report to senior administration and outside governing agencies

The ACGME recommends that all institutions provide a mechanism for reporting concerns and fears. However, even if you have a mechanism, people may still resist using it. Barriers to reporting include:

- Fear of losing support from program directors and peers

- Being labeled a tale bearer

- Fear of prejudicial treatment

- Fear of harm

Here are some recommendations for developing policies, guidelines, and procedures for confidential reporting:

- See what other institutions in your region are doing to allow residents to report and resolve conflicts in a confidential manner

- Discuss local laws and guidelines with a legal representative in your institution

- Include residents in the discussion

- Report ideas to the GMEC and administration

- Offer residents a forum to discuss a manner of reporting that feels safe and effective for them

- Write policies, guidelines, and procedures based on response with resident involvement

PROTECTING RESIDENTS' FUTURE IN MEDICAL LEGAL ISSUES

The sponsoring institution must include specifics in the initial agreement regarding liability coverage. The ACGME recommends coverage consistent with the medical staff and the institution. The residents must be covered during the training and this must include coverage for claims reported or filed after the residency period. The institution must provide proof of coverage to residents.

Important items for the institution and GMEC to address with residents include:

- Terms of coverage

- Amount of coverage

- The importance of medical record completion to malpractice cases

- Documentation ethics (e.g., avoidance of derogatory language against other providers in the records)

- Prevention of adverse events

- Statute of limitations

- Proper response to notification of a suit

- Risk management within the institution

- Moonlighting and liability coverage

- The impact of settlement decisions

- Types of available coverage (e.g., self-insurance, occurrence, claims made, claims paid, tail coverage, and nose coverage)

- What constitutes adequate coverage

Residents are less likely to be named in lawsuits than faculty attending physicians. However, every resident must be educated on liability and the impact of medical legal issues on his or her career, finances, and future decisions in practice. The institution and GMEC must commit to informing residents about liability in medicine.

AGREEMENTS WITH PARTICIPATING SITES

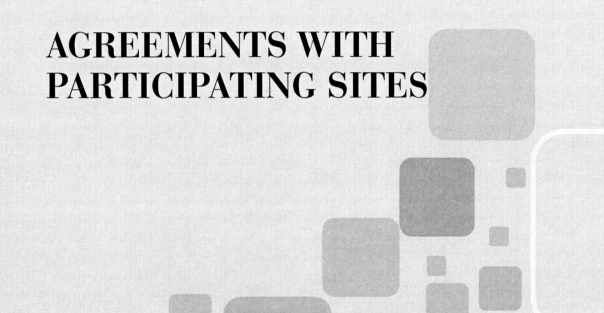

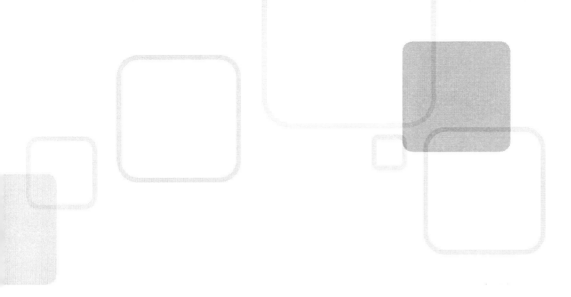

AGREEMENTS WITH PARTICIPATING SITES

The Accreditation Council for Graduate Medical Education (ACGME) requires institutions and residency programs to have legal agreements outlining the requirements and expectations of residents when rotating at institutions and sites other than the sponsoring institution. These agreements must also outline the responsibilities of the sponsoring institution and major participating institutions. There are two types of agreements:

- Master affiliation agreement for major participating institutions

- Program letter of agreement (PLA) for all participating sites

MASTER AFFILIATION AGREEMENTS

Sponsoring institutions must have master affiliation agreements with sites that are considered "major participating institutions." The ACGME defines a major participating institution as an institution that has the following characteristics:[1]

- For a two-year program, all residents in at least one program spend at least four months in a single required rotation or a combination of required rotations

- For a program of three years or longer, all residents in at least one program spend at least six months in a single required rotation or a combination of required rotations

- Programs of one-year duration are ineligible for major participating institution status

Master affiliation agreements may include the following content:

- Responsibilities of the sponsoring institution

- Responsibilities of the participating institution

- Responsibilities of the resident

- Terms of the agreement

- Liability coverage

- Institutional requirements such as compliance with the Health Insurance Portability and Accountability Act of 1996 (HIPAA), medical records completion, and compliance training

- Terms of termination

- Compensation, if applicable

- Exhibits such as copies of resident supervision policies and duty hours policies

- Compliance requirements

- Signatures of appropriate institutional officials

The content of the master agreement for major participating institutions is at the discretion of the institution and legal counsel. The ACGME requires that the master agreement be renewed at least every five years. (See an example of a master affiliation agreement for major participating institutions in Appendix 1.)

The sponsoring institution must oversee the quality of resident education when residents are rotating at participating institutions. The sponsoring institution may assign the designated institutional official (DIO) to be the liaison who communicates with the leadership at the participating institution when developing agreements. The sponsoring institution, the DIO, and the program director are responsible for educational experience, institutional compliance, and resident supervision at both the sponsoring institution and the participating institution.

The sponsoring institution may monitor the education, administration, and supervision at the participating institution by several means, including:

- Post-rotation surveys to residents asking about education, work hours, faculty accessibility during rotation period, and so forth

- Evaluation of duty hour adherence at the participating institution

- Post-rotation evaluation of residents

- Evaluation of the participating institution's resources and facilities for resident training

- Monitoring of faculty presence during surgical services similar to requirements at the sponsoring institution

The sponsoring institution must commit to oversight of resident education at participating institutions, and the participating institution must be willing to provide quality education in a safe learning environment with investment in quality patient care.

PROGRAM LETTERS OF AGREEMENT

The program director and sponsoring institution must complete a PLA with all sites where the residents rotate. (See an example of a PLA in Appendix 2.) The PLA may be shorter than the master affiliation agreement, but it must contain key elements that define the roles and responsibilities of the participating site. The program director must define the scope of training desired for the resident while at the participating site. He or she is responsible for appointing the supervising faculty at the participating site and maintaining open communication with the faculty. The program director may visit the participating site to evaluate resident responsibilities, plan a meeting with the supervising faculty at the site, and review the agreement with the leadership, supervising faculty, and program director at the site.

The agreement usually contains:

- Identification of the program director and supervising faculty at the participating site

- Responsibilities of the program director at the participating site

- Responsibilities of faculty members who will assume the educational, supervisory, and administrative roles at the participating site

- Goals and objectives of the training experience

- Responsibilities of residents while at the participating site

- The assigned rotation period

- How the residents will be evaluated

- Allotted time to complete the rotation

- Who is responsible for getting evaluation information to the sponsoring institution

- Policies and procedures that govern residents while at the participating site (e.g., resident supervision, duty hours restrictions, etc.)

- HIPAA obligations

Additional items that might be included in the PLA include:

- Institutional policies of the participating site related to resident training

- Compensation requests, if applicable

- Who will cover benefits and liability coverage during the rotation period

- Teaching faculty qualifications (which should be commensurate with the accrediting agency's faculty requirements)

- Additional compliance requirements by either the sponsoring institution or the participating site

- How resident time will be recorded

KEEPING AGREEMENTS ORGANIZED AND UP TO DATE

Similar to major affiliation agreements, PLAs must be reviewed and renewed or terminated at least every five years. The institutional agreements and PLAs must be in place during institutional reviews. Institutions may find it helpful to develop a database in an electronic system that would allow them to identify important information and dates in agreements.

Sample database fields include:

- The name of the participating institution

- The participating institution's accreditation status (e.g., changes in status since the last ACGME review, loss of accreditation, etc.)

- The name of the program and service on which the resident is rotating

- The program accreditation status

- The type of agreement (e.g., master affiliation agreement or PLA)

- The date the agreement is initiated

- The duration of the agreement

- The renewal dates of the agreement, if continuous

- The program or service requesting agreement

Working collaboratively with your institution's legal team can be helpful in organizing this database. The legal team and graduate medical education (GME) leaders collaboratively can decide on the best dates to initiate and terminate agreements, based on the needs of the GME office and the sponsoring institution, and other service agreements within the institution. They can also decide on an identification labeling system that will allow for easy retrieval of agreements across the institution. A collaborative approach allows for better communication regarding content and important dates for agreements.

Additionally, institutions might elect to review agreements during two important periods:

- During each program's internal review process

- Annually, when programs submit residents' rotation schedules for the academic year

ENDNOTES

1. ACGME. August 2007. "Frequently Asked Questions Related to Master Affiliation Agreements and Program Letters of Agreement." *www.acgme.org/acWebsite/about/ab_FAQAgreement.pdf.*

THE INTERNAL REVIEW

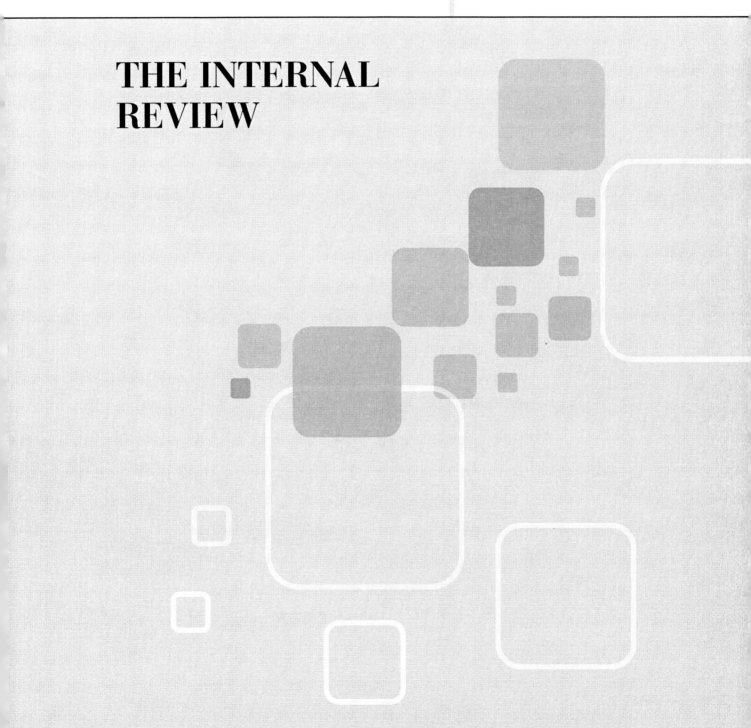

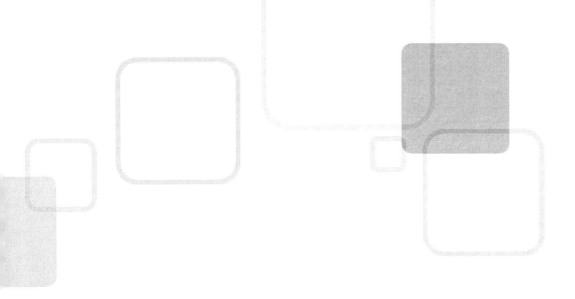

THE INTERNAL REVIEW

The internal review is a structured internal evaluation of graduate medical education (GME) programs. The Accreditation Council for Graduate Medical Education (ACGME) requires sponsoring institutions to conduct an internal review in the middle of their accreditation cycles.

The purpose of the internal review is to evaluate educational programs, curricula, resident performance, procedures, resources, and support systems. During the internal review, you should also evaluate that program's compliance with the institutional requirements, common program requirements, and program-specific requirements of the ACGME. In addition, the review process evaluates the program's advancement in areas of faculty development and resident achievement on certification exams.

The internal review process is planned, organized, and implemented under the leadership of the graduate medical education committee (GMEC). It is designed to evaluate programs prior to the residency review committee (RRC) site visit. The aggregate information received from all of the programs in the institution during the internal review can be helpful in identifying those areas that need improvement prior to the institutional review. During the institutional review, the ACGME field staff reviewer will evaluate the institutional process for the internal review, the membership on the internal review committee for each program's internal review, and the protocol used by the institution to conduct the internal review. Each internal review is an opportune time for the sponsoring institution to reassess before the institutional review.

KEY COMPONENTS

The internal review protocol should include:

- **Selection of the internal review committee for each program:** The GMEC selects the members of the internal review committee. The ACGME recommends at least one resident and one faculty member, each from a different GME program in the sponsoring institution, with options for other members from other programs in the sponsoring institution or an outside institution. Additional reviewers might include administrators, residents, and educators within the sponsoring institution, and faculty or administrators from other participating institutions and programs.

- **Explanation of cycle time and when internal review is scheduled:** The cycle time is defined as the time from the last accreditation to the next expected visit. The internal review must be scheduled approximately midway between the accreditation and the site visit. Although exact dates are not necessary, the ACGME does require that you attempt to schedule and conduct the internal review near the midway point.

- **Review of important documents:** Each member of the internal review committee must review the CPRs and the program-specific requirements for the program being evaluated. Additionally, the designated institutional official (DIO) might develop questions for the internal review that address program support, financial resources, educational activities and monitoring, compliance, ACGME competencies, and other resident and faculty performance measures. The committee members must review questions that are to be used during the process before the actual interviews and the inquiry into records. Committee members should also review accreditation letters from previous ACGME visits and reviews, responses from resident surveys, and previous program evaluations. The ACGME will not review every document used in the internal review during the institutional review. However, the field staff reviewer will want to know that the institution has a protocol to evaluate programs effectively and that the institution has a standard structure for scheduling the review. The Internal Review Document (IRD) will ask about membership selection for the internal review committee to confirm appropriate representation. The field staff reviewer will confirm these items with the program directors and the DIO during the institutional site visit. (See Figure 5.1 for a list of helpful documents.)

FIGURE 5.1

Helpful documents for your internal review

Regardless of the institutional protocol for the internal review, the review committee will need several documents to get answers for the inquiry during the process. Here is a list of potential documents that might be helpful during the internal review:

- Documentation of faculty responsible for teaching and research within the program and at participating sites
- Resident information (e.g., the number of residents in each postgraduate year [PGY] level, demographics, etc.)
- The names and number of programs within the department
- The names of leaders responsible for educating and evaluating residents
- Accreditation status and date
- The date of the last review
- Any previous citations
- Actions taken to correct citations
- A description of support from the sponsoring institution, chair, and other institutions
- A list of staff support and responsibilities
- A summary of resident responsibilities
- A description of the curriculum for each PGY level
- The methods used to evaluate residents and the faculty
- Documentation that the educational curriculum and evaluation process conform to ACGME competencies
- Handbooks and manuals distributed to residents and faculty
- Policies and procedures specific to residents and the program and department (e.g., leave policies)
- Documentation of resident schedules
- A list of affiliation agreements and examples of those agreements
- Up-to-date affiliation agreements
- Documentation of accomplished compliance measures
- A scholarly activity report
- Any additional documents that demonstrate institutional, faculty, and staff commitment to the training of residents in the institution

- **Documentation of the internal review in GMEC minutes:** The GMEC minutes must reflect the timing of the internal review. The minutes should note the date the internal review is scheduled or planned, the date the review is conducted, the date of the report to the GMEC, and the date the internal review is approved by the GMEC. During the institutional review, the ACGME field staff representative will confirm that internal reviews are scheduled and in process during the expected time.

- **Evaluation of program effectiveness in meeting competencies and outcome measures:** The DIO and GMEC must develop a procedure to measure the program's effectiveness in teaching and measuring outcomes of the ACGME competencies. The institution must also have a mechanism in place to monitor program response to previous recommendations by the GMEC and response to previous citations.

THE VALUE OF CRITICAL ASSESSMENT

The internal review requires critical assessment of the individual programs and its support from the institution. The results of the program-specific reviews provide vital information that the institution can use to prepare for the institutional review. This evaluation will assist the institution, GMEC, and DIO in identifying the following:

- A protocol that does not capture the necessary measures of the ACGME competencies

- Undocumented educational outcomes

- Progress on response to GMEC recommendations and citations

- Resource needs

- Opportunities to enhance the training environment

- Compliance issues

Any issues or concerns identified during the internal review must be addressed and reported to the GMEC. The GMEC must monitor the program response and plans for corrective action. The GMEC may recommend additional modifications, additions, and corrective actions. The results of the internal review must be discussed at a GMEC meeting. Like the ACGME review, the internal review will evaluate:

- Compliance with ACGME guidelines

- Support of the sponsoring institution

- Program efforts to answer previous citations and improvements

- The effectiveness of evaluation tools (e.g., program, resident, and faculty evaluation forms)

- Evidence of quality programs and educational activities that meet the goals and objectives of the department and institution

- All materials previously submitted to the RRC

- Affiliation agreements

- Program evidence of resident education covering competency measures

- Evidence of faculty development for GME faculty and program directors

- Written policies for resident eligibility, selection, appointments, advancement, probation, and dismissal

- Written policies for the grievance and fair hearing process

- A process for measuring ACGME competencies in programs and educational activities

THE INTERNAL REVIEW REPORT

The DIO and GMEC must develop a protocol to report program growth, responses to recommended corrective action, continued concerns, and progress since the last internal review or site visit. The committee must submit a written report to the GMEC describing its findings and noted recommendations and citations.

The report should include:

- Names of the committee members

- Documentation, including the date, that the review process was completed

- Responses to questions asked during the review

- A summarized program evaluation

- A summary of residents' performance

- A summary of faculty achievements and development

- A summary of the institutional support

- Any major changes in the program's curriculum, faculty, staff, or resident number since the last review or last accreditation visit

- A summary of the educational and program quality

The internal review is a vital part of program evaluation. The sponsoring institution has a major role in developing the protocol for the internal review. The ACGME field staff reviewer will want to confirm that a process is in place at the institution to gather pertinent information for program success.

FIGURE 5.2

Institutional checklist

❏ Review institutional requirements, institutional review document, common program requirements, and program specific requirements

❏ Check accreditation of sponsoring institution and participating institutions

❏ Secure written commitment statement of sponsoring institution

❏ Identify key GME leaders

❏ Identify designee to sign important documents that must be submitted to ACGME in absence of DIO

❏ Verify institutional support to GME (i.e. financial, resources, space, technology etc.)

❏ Verify protected time of DIO, program directors, and key GME leadership

❏ Review resident rotation schedules

❏ Confirm program letters of agreements for rotations

❏ Confirm master affiliation agreements for major participating sites

❏ Review and update required written policies

❏ Verify financial support for residents

❏ Check agreement of appointment for required components

❏ Check current professional liability policy of residents for required components

❏ Collect duty hour reports from programs

❏ Check availability of resident counseling services

❏ Review availability of resident confidential reporting for concerns and exchange of information

❏ Check adequacy of ancillary support services

❏ Check availability of resident food services, call rooms, and safety

❏ Review GMEC composition, function, and reporting lines

❏ Verify adequate communication between GMEC, institution, medical staff and program director

❏ Check annual report for required elements and appropriate reporting

❏ Verify internal review occurred mid-way between last accreditation visit and next site visit

❏ Check internal review report for ACGME required elements

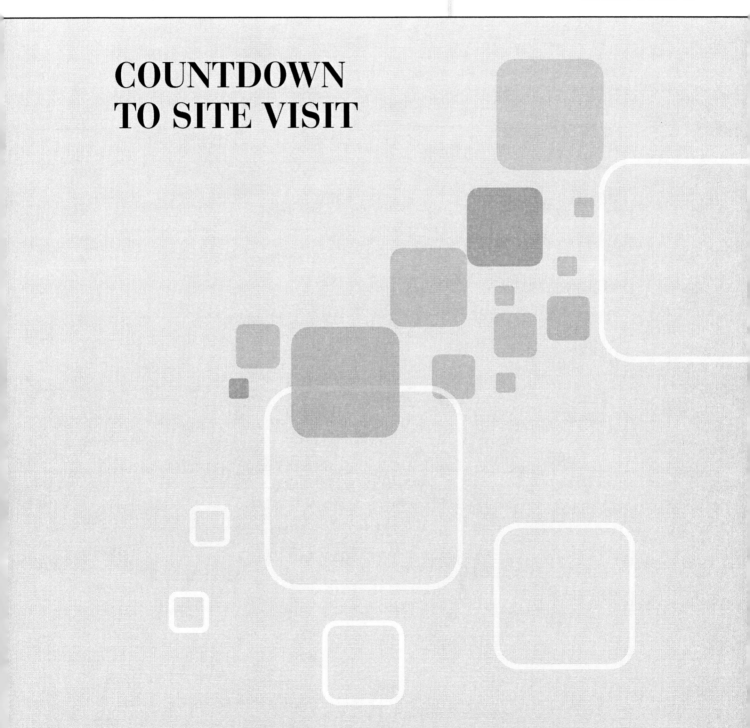

COUNTDOWN
TO SITE VISIT

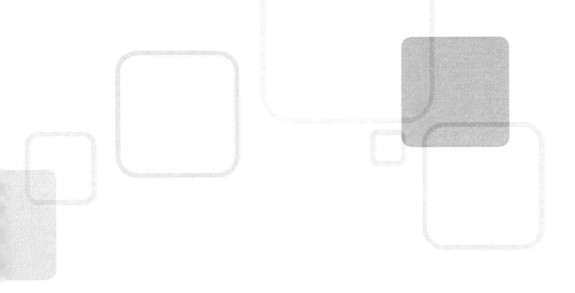

COUNTDOWN TO SITE VISIT

Preparing for an Accreditation Council for Graduation Medical Education (ACGME) institutional review adds a great deal of work to your daily responsibilities. It is daunting, to be sure, but you should try to approach it with a positive attitude. Remember, this could be a great opportunity for your institution's graduate medical education (GME) programs to shine. This is also an opportunity to find out where any weaknesses are—and fix them.

TWENTY-FOUR MONTHS BEFORE REVIEW

STEP 1: ESTABLISH A TIMELINE

At least two years before the institutional review, begin to develop a schedule to ensure that you have ample time to gather the needed information. The ACGME institutional site visit is a structured evaluation, and it's important to be prepared. Working backward, set dates for:

- Completing the ACGME institutional review document (IRD)

- Gathering pertinent documents that must be attached to the IRD (look at the field staff documentation checklist at the end of the IRD)

- Creating a list of the citations received by each residency program at its most recent accreditation visit

- Securing a signed commitment from the institutional officials in support of GME

- Updating key policies (e.g., resident eligibility and selection, resident supervision, disaster policy, vendor policy, etc.)

- Reviewing the resident agreement of appointment to ensure that all required components are present

- Updating the organizational chart

- Reviewing the report given to the medical staff and participating institutions for required components

- Reviewing details—including ACGME institutional requirements (IRs), common program requirements (CPRs), and your institution's responses on the IRD—with people who may be interviewed by the ACGME field reviewer

- Ensuring that key people understand the structure and function of the graduate medical education committee (GMEC) and that they will have no problem answering questions from the field reviewer

It is important to begin early with the preparation process and be realistic about how long each task will take. You know what response time is like in your organization. If response time is long, consider starting more than two years before the review.

STEP 2: GET FAMILIAR WITH THE IRD

The ACGME's IRD provides a good guide for the steps you need to take to prepare for the institutional review. The IRD is a two-part document. You can download IRD—Part I from the ACGME Accreditation Data System (ADS), which is on the Web at *https://www.acgme.org/ads/default.asp*. (Sponsoring institutions receive a user ID and password to access the ADS.) When you download Part I from the Web site, it is already complete. Part I contains identifying information of the sponsoring institution, major participating institutions, and the designated institutional official (DIO). Part I also lists the number of accredited programs the ACGME has documented for the sponsoring institution, including the number of filled positions. In Part I, the DIO will also find the list of programs with accreditation status and the recommended dates of the internal review. The fourth section contains the response to previous citations in the sponsoring institution.

You can download IRD—Part II directly from the Web at *www.acgme.org/acWebsite/navPages/nav_IRC.asp*. The DIO verifies and updates Part I annually. IRD—Part II must be submitted right before the institutional review. Plan to mail Part II about a month in advance of the review, just to make sure it gets there in plenty of time.

IRD—Part II has very specific instructions. Read through the entire document before starting to answer the questions contained therein. There are three checklists at the end of IRD—Part II: the Field Staff Documentation Checklist, Attachment Checklist, and Completion Checklist. It's a good idea to review these checklists and keep them handy as you prepare for the review. You must also submit these checklists as part of IRD—Part II. (For the remainder of this chapter, "IRD" will refer to Part II, unless otherwise noted.)

STEP 3: REVIEW CITATIONS

You should think about citations very early in the preparation process. You can find a list of common citations on the Institutional Review page of the ACGME Web site (*www.acgme.org/acWebsite/navPages/nav_IRC.asp*). Since these citations are common, this is something the ACGME field reviewer is likely to be looking for during your institutional review. So, you'll want to double-check those areas to make sure your institution is in compliance.

Next, review the previous citations your institution has received. Review both institutional citations and program-specific citations. Checking these areas at least two years in advance allows time to correct any remaining deficiencies and improve upon new processes that are in the early stages of correction.

TWENTY-TWO MONTHS BEFORE REVIEW

STEP 4: CREATE YOUR REVIEW PREP TEAM

The next step in the preparation stage is to create a team that will assist in gathering information, identifying missing documents, writing policies and guidelines, identifying missing procedures, and openly giving a critical, constructive assessment of the status of the sponsoring institution.

The review prep team should:

- Present an initial institutional overview of its findings from program documents, institutional documents, and team evaluations to the DIO and GMEC. The summary report will call attention to those items within the institution that are a priority for a successful institutional review but currently are being overlooked.

- Discuss the institutional review with key administration in the sponsoring institution.

- Review initial plans for corrective action of program citations.

- Report to the DIO and GMEC the status of corrective action plans, including whether the actions were initiated, citations were resolved, and outcome measures were established.

- Discuss action plans for correcting unresolved citations before the IRD is due.

- Discuss concerns about policies and procedures, institutional support, facilities, and GME flow and processes.

- Know the institution's strengths and weaknesses.

STEP 5: UPDATE IRD—PART I

Now, look at the information currently in IRD—Part I regarding the sponsoring institution and major participating institutions. Ask each program director whether he or she has reported new major participating sites to the residency review committee (RRC) and the institution's DIO. If the information supplied in Part I is incorrect, notify the DIO, who must report the information to the ACGME. The corrections to Part I must be submitted online, as outlined in the IRD instructions. The DIO must review and verify the information in Part I.

EIGHTEEN MONTHS BEFORE REVIEW

STEP 6: STUDY IRD—PART II

Completing the IRD will take a good deal of time. Consider dividing the IRD sections among the review prep team members. Start by gathering the team to read through the IRD and the three checklists at the end. As you do so, identify key materials needed to begin the documentation process.

Team members can gather different information and write responses. However, at the end of the process, the DIO or his or her designee will put all of the information into the IRD form. The IRD form is a Microsoft Word document, and the instructions clearly state that you should submit the information only through this particular form. The person completing the final form should be proficient with Microsoft Word. He or she must follow the directions *exactly as outlined* in the document, *in the exact order*, and *place attachments at the end of the document as instructed in sequential order*. The document alert states that attachments are not needed for all items, and responses should fit in the given spaces. Be careful to include all information requested, and number pages consecutively as directed for all attachments. This is very important, as failure to follow the instructions exactly may result in a citation.

During the review, the ACGME field staff will confirm the information provided in the IRD through interviews with key leaders in the sponsoring institution, GME administration, the DIO, program directors, GMEC members, residents, and related staff members. The field reviewer will also ask to see various documents, such as policies and procedures. The gray boxes on the IRD identify the main information to prepare for the review. Keep in mind, though, that the inquiry and review are not limited to the information listed in the IRD. Make sure to have plenty of supporting documents readily available for review.

FOURTEEN MONTHS BEFORE THE REVIEW

STEP 7: COMPLETE SECTION 5 OF THE IRD

Section 5 is the first section you need to complete in the IRD. (Sections 1-4 are in IRD—Part I.) This section focuses on the institutional organization and responsibilities. It covers four areas:

- The sponsoring institution

- The institution's commitment to GME

- Institutional agreements

- Accreditation for patient care in sponsoring hospitals and major participating hospital sites.

Describing the sponsoring institution

The first question on the IRD asks for a description of the sponsoring institution. Keep in mind that each residency program can have only one sponsoring institution that is responsible for the quality and maintenance of the educational experience and for the quality of patient care. Each person participating in the institutional review and all staff members, program directors, administration, and residents must be familiar with the institution's mission, goals, and objectives for patient care, and its goals and objectives for GME.

The person completing the IRD and those interviewed by the ACGME field staff must be familiar with the sponsoring institution's organizational structure and reporting lines, the structural and functional model of education, medical school affiliations, academic partnerships, and multi-institutional consortia memberships. They should also understand the history and important characteristics of the sponsoring institution, and how the leadership accentuates the learning environment and its uniqueness. The information must be sufficient to complete the paragraph on the sponsoring institution.

The ACGME also asks that any changes since the last institutional review affecting GME programs be reported on the IRD. Report the following changes:

- New institutional leaders (e.g., CEO or CMO)

- Newly appointed academic leadership such as a new dean, vice president, or chancellor

- A decrease in institutional funding support for educational programs

- A new board of managers whose point of view regarding the distribution of training support may be different from that of previous managers

- A change in institutional directions regarding specific GME programs

Program-specific citations

Next, the IRD asks about program-specific citations. It instructs the institution to refer to IRD— Part I and describe corrective actions taken in response to institutional citations. The DIO and GMEC should outline steps taken to address citations and any recent responses or progress reports.

The IRD requests that the institution supply information to program-specific citations on Attachment I of the IRD. Documentation includes citation categories that every program sponsored by the institution has received. The Attachment 1 form, included at the end of IRD—Part II, is designed to list program-specific citations organized into six categories. The IRD Attachment 1 citation category document represents specific program citations that require tighter oversight by the sponsoring institution and areas that the DIO and GMEC must focus on to meet ACGME compliance. During the institutional review, the ACGME field staff will assess actions taken by the sponsoring institution and programs to resolve listed citations.

Attachment 2 must contain the actions taken to address citations received on the most recent program site visit. The response must be placed in categories demonstrated on Attachment I. The sponsoring institution and program must demonstrate a collaborative effort to correct citations and show how the results of the corrective action will be measured. Program-specific citations and corrective action may be reported in several formats. The key point is to keep information concise and organized by citation category.

Take the following steps to prepare Attachments 1 and 2:

1. Review program RRC letters to assess citations from the most recent program review.

2. Document the programs adjacent to the appropriate citation categories listed as represented on Attachment 1.

3. Have the DIO and GMEC review and make recommendations to programs regarding corrective actions for the program citations if not already resolved since the last RRC review.

4. Assess programs for resolution of citations.

5. Describe the sponsoring institution's and program's action in addressing corrective actions for program citations (Attachment 2).

6. List the outcome measures (Attachment 2).

For examples of corrective actions and outcome measures, see Figure 6.1. See Figures 6.2 and 6.3 for templates on organization information related to accreditation, citations, and corrective action.

During early preparation for the institutional review, all citations that programs have not addressed should be discussed at a GMEC meeting or with the DIO to evaluate barriers to progress and reevaluate the timeline for corrective action.

The ACGME field staff reviewer will ask to see evidence of progress and outcome measures during the institutional review. The field staff reviewer will also request verification of participation of the sponsoring institution in resolving noncompliance. The DIO must be actively involved in organizing and developing the guidelines for monitoring corrective actions in the programs and the sponsoring institution.

FIGURE 6.1

Examples of solutions to citations

EXAMPLE 1

Citation: lack of commitment of sponsoring institution

Corrective actions:

- Discuss citation and concerns with departmental chair, program director, and key administrative leaders
- Ask the sponsoring institution to recommend an administrative partner who can attend GMEC meetings on a regular basis and meet with the DIO and key GME leaders to discuss special concerns regularly
- Work together to outline ways the sponsoring institution can increase support for the GME program, such as increase funding for technology, develop solutions to meet manpower needs without compromising duty hours, increase the number of faculty members to meet instruction and supervision needs, and assist with quality measures of resident care
- Discuss who will be responsible for carrying out these plans and negotiating changes

Outcome measures:

- The budget is increased to meet the program's technology needs
- Duty hours are monitored and evaluated, especially in areas at risk for noncompliance with regulations
- Faculty members are hired to meet the faculty-to-resident ratio that is needed to provide appropriate supervision and instruction

EXAMPLE 2

Citation: no documentation of resident supervision in the operating room

Corrective actions:

- Review the policy and guidelines for resident supervision with the GMEC, administrators of the sponsoring institution, the medical staff, the program director, and residents
- Discuss details of institutional policies, including the function of the sponsoring institution in setting standards, procedures for monitoring, and fostering compliance with guidelines
- Meet with the quality officer to develop a monitoring protocol
- Present to medical staff members, administrators, program directors, and residents the consequences of noncompliance
- Review the progress report quarterly for evidence of improvement

Outcome measures:

- An improvement in the time to perform OR cases with an attending present
- The overall culture change among the medical staff and faculty
- A documented increase in attending physician presence in the OR

FIGURE 6.2

Example of template for assessment of citations and proposed corrective actions for sponsoring institution and participating institutions

	Date of last ACGME review	Citation category	Resolved (Y/N)	Barriers to completion	Date of internal review	Citation category	Resolved (Y/N)
Sponsoring institution		**Citation(s): did not schedule internal review midway between program site visits. Pediatrics (I.1)** **Corrective action(s):** 1. Check for the date of the next program review of remaining programs. 2. Schedule an internal review if midway. 3. Develop a reminder system. **GMEC** 1. Consider an electronic reminder system. 2. Schedule at the time of program review with interval reminders. **Outcome measure(s):** All remaining programs have an internal review at the appropriate time.				**Citation(s):** **Corrective action(s):** **GMEC recommendation(s):** **Outcome measure(s):**	
Major participating institution		(Those related to resident education) **Citation(s):** **Corrective action(s):** **GMEC recommendation(s):** **Outcome measure(s):**					

FIGURE 6.3

Assessment of accreditation of sponsoring institution and participating institutions specific to program

	Date of last RRC review	Citations	Resolved (Y/N)	Date of internal review	Citations
Family Medicine		Citation(s): Corrective action(s): GMEC and institution recommendation(s): Outcome measure(s):			Citation(s): Corrective action(s): GMEC and institution recommendation(s): Outcome measure(s):
General Surgery		Citation(s): Corrective action(s): GMEC and institution recommendation(s): Outcome measure(s):			Citation(s): Corrective action(s): GMEC and institution recommendation(s): Outcome measure(s):

It is important for the DIO or main person filing the IRD to have available a hard copy or some form of documentation of all accreditation letters for the sponsoring institution (i.e., GME accreditation and patient care accreditation), participating institutions, and programs; all program-specific reviews including citations; and all letters sent to ACGME and/or RRCs to address concerns and citations. These items are helpful during the field staff visit.

Describing the sponsoring institution's commitment to GME

The next questions on the IRD have to do with the sponsoring institution's commitment to GME. GME commitment is measured in several ways, including the sponsoring institution's oversight of GME programs and its hiring of appropriate faculty and administrative leaders to maintain both hospital accreditation and GME accreditation. On the IRD, you need to demonstrate that the sponsoring institution has resources, policies and procedures, and personnel in place to promote residents' professional, ethical, and personal development. You also need to describe how the sponsoring institution supports safe and appropriate patient care within its GME programs. Furthermore, you must show that the sponsoring institution collaborates with the GMEC, the

GME office, and individual GME programs to provide appropriate resources and activities. The ACGME field staff reviewer will confirm these resources and activities during the institutional review through interviews with the DIO, GMEC members, GME representatives, residents, and medical staff leadership. The IRD requests examples of at least two activities that demonstrate the institution's commitment to GME and two activities that demonstrate commitment to patient safety.

In addition to describing activities that represent the sponsoring institution's commitment to GME, you must also attach the institution's statement of commitment to GME as Attachment 3. (See a sample statement of commitment in Figure 6.4.) This statement of commitment must have been signed and dated by the institution's governance, administration, and GME leadership within the past year.

Also under *Commitment to GME* on the IRD, you must provide the following information:

- The institutional reporting relationship for GME, including an organizational chart as Attachment 4 (see Figure 2.1 in Chapter 2 for a sample organizational chart)

- Confirmation that a system is in place to ensure that the DIO or a designee reviews and cosigns all information submitted to ACGME by program directors

- A description of GME annual reports including a description of content, who gives them, how they are given, and to whom they are given

- The amount of the DIO's time that is allocated to GME responsibilities

- Resources provided to the GME office, programs, residents, and staff members, including technology, salary support, educational materials, space, protected time, and more

- Confirmation of an institutional disaster policy, which should be included as Attachment 5

During the review, make sure to have evidence of these areas of support on hand to show the ACGME field staff members. For example, you might want to have a copy of the latest annual report, the DIO's job description, and a written policy regarding the DIO's or designee's approval of all submissions to the ACGME.

FIGURE 6.4

Example of commitment between sponsoring institution and medical education

Annotated areas include Committee to promote professionalism, ethical behavior, and quality patient care; Committee reporting structure in the sponsoring institution.

Graduate Medical Education Mission Statement

The Department of Medical Education creates high quality medical educational experiences that lead to the development of excellent Physicians, and extraordinary Healthcare Leaders.

Our Global Commitment to Medical Education

The efforts of the sponsoring institution are aligned with the GME Mission to enhance the health of the individuals in the institution catchment area and surrounding communities through the following commitments: (1) advancing medical education through innovative curricula; (2) pursuit of scholarly activity; and (3) support of evidence-based community-oriented research to train the next generation of professional healthcare leaders and health care providers.

In accordance with accrediting agencies and maintaining the Medical Education programs of this institution, we commit to providing high quality evidence-based medical education with the following goals:

- To provide quality patient care that is compassionate, appropriate, and effective;
- To provide adequate resources and facilities for exemplary learning and patient care;
- To provide esteemed faculty and leaders for medical education;
- To promote culturally sensitive practice-based learning and improvement;
- To appraise and assimilate scientific evidence;
- To use empathetic interpersonal and communication skills with patients, their families, colleagues, and co-workers;
- To commit to accountability with professional responsibilities;
- To commit to oversight of all medical education training programs;
- To adhere to values and character of high ethical and moral principles;
- To teach a systematic approach to learning and implementing healthcare "best practice" models;
- To pursue opportunities to train healthcare professionals in the advancement of medical innovations.
- Being community educators and leaders.

In pursuit of these goals, the sponsoring institution provides Medical Education programs that are valuable and unique to other training programs in being balanced in education and service, comprehensive, and patient centered.

Resources

One of the most important ways the sponsoring institution demonstrates its commitment to GME is through the resources it provides. The ACGME field staff is likely to spend a lot of time on this during the review. GME programs cannot function without adequate financial resources, medical education materials, technology, library support, and institutional staffing support to meet demands for structured learning. The sponsoring institution must be able to demonstrate that it is providing necessary resources or partnering with an academic affiliate to share educational resources.

SIX MONTHS BEFORE VISIT

Demonstrating institutional agreements

The next important activity is to assess all program reviews, rotation schedules, and affiliation agreements for accuracy and renewal dates. All agreements must be reviewed a minimum of every five years.

On the IRD, you must describe how the sponsoring institution oversees and monitors the quality of GME at its own and participating sites. For examples of effective ways to do this, see Chapter 4.

Important information to have available during institutional review includes:

- The most recent rotation schedule for all of the programs in your institution (be sure to verify them with the tracking systems in your institution, as well as with residents and program directors)

- A list of all the program letters of agreement (PLAs) for all sites where residents are rotating for each program sponsored by your institution, as well as copies of the actual PLAs

- A list of all master affiliation agreements with major participating institutions, as well as copies of the actual agreements

- Renewal dates for agreements

- A sample of a major affiliation agreement format (see an example in Appendix 1)

Note: Plan to review agreement details at least annually to make sure all elements are present and the program directors' rotation rosters match the agreements.

It is important to have quick access to this information during the institutional review. (For examples of effective ways to store and file agreements and pertinent materials, see Chapter 4.)

FIVE MONTHS BEFORE VISIT

Proving accreditation

When renewing agreements make sure all major participating institutions and program affiliations have met accreditation requirements. The field reviewer will confirm the accreditation during the site visit.

STEP 8: COMPLETE SECTION 6 OF THE IRD

Section 6 is the second section you need to complete in the IRD. This section focuses on the sponsoring institution's responsibilities to residents. It covers six areas:

- Eligibility and selection of residents

- Financial support for residents

- Benefits and conditions of appointment

- Agreement of appointment

- Resident participation in educational and professional activities

- Resident educational and work environment

Overview: Institutional responsibilities to residents

As you prepare for the review, you need to ensure that the sponsoring institution is meeting its responsibilities to residents. The ACGME mandates that the sponsoring institution outline its responsibilities to residents both in a commitment document and in information provided to residents before employment and throughout the resident education period. During the review, your team should demonstrate that the sponsoring institution has provided written policies and guidelines to inform residents of procedures and to ensure that residents receive a quality education and a safe work environment within the institution. Policies and guidelines must be updated and shared with residents as outlined by your institutional bylaws and governing agencies.

Examples of communication with residents include the following:

- Have regular meetings with chief residents to review and discuss current policies and guidelines

- Have chief residents convey information to their colleagues at departmental meetings

- Work with resident representatives on committees to develop ways to optimize sharing of information

- Publish new policies and recommendations in institutional newsletters

- Publish a resident manual that contains pertinent guidelines and policies and disperse it to residents annually

- Plan information or training sessions to review the most important policy changes

Showing compliance with resident-related requirements

The ACGME field staff will review the written policies and procedures for resident eligibility and selection. The policy serves as a guideline to prevent discriminatory hiring practices. The field staff will also look at the financial support the institution provides to residents. He or she will confirm that the support is adequate to allow the residents to fulfill their educational responsibilities through interviews with residents and others during the review. In addition, the institution must show that candidates for resident positions are informed of the terms, conditions, and benefits of appointment.

Institutional commitments must be presented in the resident's initial contract agreement of appointment, in policies, and in resident manuals. Some institutions may prefer to have all material in a contractual agreement and others may prefer to present it in multiple formats. The ACGME lists several required elements for the agreement of appointment. The institution must document on the IRD that these elements are included in their standard agreement of appointment for residents. You must also prepare an annotated copy of the contractual agreement, which the ACGME field staff will look at on the day of the review. When completing the IRD section on agreement details, remember to check either the "yes" or the "no" box. Only "no" answers require explanation.

Demonstrating resident participation

Your team will need to demonstrate that residents are actively participating in professional committees and educational programs. The sponsoring institution must list on the IRD those committees and councils that allow resident participation. The institution must also demonstrate its role in monitoring resident participation on committees and educational programs for outcomes in the ACGME competencies. Resident membership on committees and councils must be included with the IRD as Attachment 6.

Describing the resident educational and work environment

Rapport with residents is important when making decisions that might affect program accreditation, institutional accreditation, and work environment policies and guidelines. During the review, the ACGME will want to see that the sponsoring institution and GMEC have developed a mechanism for residents to report concerns or potential risks. These concerns may be reviewed in committee meetings, but it is important to have an opportunity for confidential reporting. Many states have guidelines and laws regarding confidential reporting when it relates to patient safety, unsafe work environments, and potential risk regarding employment.

The institutional review will cover several areas regarding the residents' work and educational environment, including patient support services, medical records, food services for residents, on-call rooms/sleeping quarters for residents, and personal safety and security.

Reviewing institutional policies on a regular basis is important to ensure that resident-related issues are included in the policies and to assess the need for GME-specific policies. Each institution will have hospital-specific procedures for developing, writing, and posting policies and guidelines. The sponsoring institution will also have policies that are pertinent to all employees, including residents. The sponsoring institution, administration, GMEC, and DIO can work collaboratively to review policies and coordinate details to meet the requirements of the institution, the governing bodies, and the GME accrediting organizations. (See Table 1.1 in Chapter 1 for required and suggested policies and guidelines.) The field staff reviewer will check for written policies on topics such as harassment and employing residents with disabilities.

The field staff reviewer will speak with residents during the review and look at the results of the resident survey. All information reported to the ACGME, including the IRD, attachments, resident survey, and interviews with other institutional and program personnel, is potential material that could be discussed with residents. These items include, but are not limited to:

- Organizational structure

- Reporting lines of institution

- Resident agreement contents

- Location and content of facility resources

- Information about financial commitment

- Resident education and evaluation methods

- Faculty participation in training

- Facility resources

- Safe work environments

As you prepare for the institutional review, take time to go over these types of issues with residents. They need to have a thorough understanding of all policies, procedures, and operations throughout the institution.

THREE MONTHS BEFORE REVIEW

STEP 9: COMPLETE SECTION 7 OF THE IRD

Section 7 is the third section you need to complete in the IRD. This section focuses on the GMEC. It covers two areas:

- GMEC composition and meetings

- GMEC responsibilities

GMEC requirements

In this phase of preparation, it's important to assess the GMEC to make sure its composition and functions meet the ACGME requirements, as discussed in Chapter 1. On the IRD, you'll need to confirm that the institution meets the requirements or you must explain why it doesn't. You must also describe the operating structure of your institution's GMEC. All faculty, residents, medical staff members, GME officials, and institutional officials must know the function of the GMEC. The institution must be aware of the subcommittees, any executive committees, and other involvements from consortia, major participating institutions, and any dual accreditations where applicable.

These items are important for the IRD:

- Check the membership roster to be sure it includes the DIO, peer-nominated residents, program directors, and GME administrators. You must include a list of current members as Attachment 7.

- Confirm the standing meeting time and place for the GMEC. Document that the meeting occurs at least quarterly.

- Assess the GMEC meeting minutes to make sure important elements are recorded, as outlined by the ACGME. The minutes from each GMEC meeting held over the past 12 months must be included with the IRD as Attachment 8. The minutes of two meetings must be highlighted to document required GMEC actions.

The ACGME spells out many responsibilities for the GMEC in its IRs. The IRD asks the institution to document compliance with each GMEC responsibility. It also requires that an institutional policy—one regarding interactions between vendors and residents/GME programs—be submitted as Attachment 9.

It may be helpful for you to make a checklist of GMEC functions. Consider also creating an institutional document outlining GMEC functions and institutional support to carry out those functions. (See the checklist in Figure 6.5.)

FIGURE 6.5

GMEC checklist

The sponsoring institution must document that the GMEC carries out the following responsibilities:

☒ Negotiate with sponsoring institution for resident stipends, benefits, and resources
☒ Develop a communication forum for program directors to communicate with participating sites
☒ Develop and implement policies and procedures related to resident governance, education, compliance, supervision, and duty hours
☒ Review all accreditation letters after program site visit
☒ Approve important information before forwarding to ACGME

STEP 10: COMPLETE SECTION 8 OF THE IRD

Section 8 is the fourth and final section you need to complete in the IRD. This section focuses on the internal review. It covers two areas:

- Internal review process

- Internal review report

Internal review

The internal review is a time not only for program internal review, but also for assessment of sponsoring institution support for each specific residency program and residency education as a whole. Internal review documents must demonstrate that at least one faculty member and one resident from a program other than the program being reviewed is included in the review.

When preparing to complete this section of the IRD, take the following steps:

- Clearly outline the internal review protocol and include it as Attachment 10.

- Check your internal reviews to see whether they were conducted according to these guidelines (and if not, make a note to correct that in future reviews).

- Make sure the DIO and program directors fully understand the procedures for internal review.

- Make sure the date of internal review reported to the ACGME Part I ADS and the date recorded on this internal review report regarding each program matches the date on the internal review for each program. The ACGME gives three options for selecting the "date of the internal review" that will be used for documentation. The DIO should determine which option the institution will use in dating the internal review to avoid discrepancies.

- Go over RRC reviews, letters accompanying each review, and internal review reports, and include these reports for each program as Attachment 11.

This is a great opportunity to assess your process for internal review. Also consider interval reports for those programs that have RRC citations that were not addressed at the time of the internal review.

ONE MONTH BEFORE REVIEW

STEP 11: FINALIZING AND MAILING THE IRD

Your team should be just about ready to send its IRD and supporting attachments to the ACGME. You need to mail them well in advance of the review, but before submitting the documents, make sure the following tasks are complete:

- The DIO has signed page 1 of the IRD

- All IRD formatting, including the numbering of pages and placement of attachments, is in accordance with the ACGME IRD completion checklist and instructions

- All answers on the IRD have been reviewed and verified by the DIO, GMEC, institutional representative(s), program directors, residents, and supporting staff members

- IRD instructions have been followed, including those regarding recommended paper size, order of pagination, tabs and dividers, and attachments

TWO WEEKS BEFORE THE REVIEW

STEP 12: FINAL PREPARATIONS

Prior to the institutional site visit, the DIO will arrange the time and date with the ACGME. The institutional key administrative representatives, staff, and DIO should review schedules and dates within the institution to avoid conflicting schedules, absences of key personnel, and overlapping major institutional events.

Review all documents, including the IRD and attachments, with the GMEC, residents, program directors, and anyone who could be interviewed.

The DIO and preparation team must make sure all documents previously submitted are available for review during the site visit. The field reviewer will also want to see policies, guidelines, examples of agreements, institutional policies, evidence of collaboration, and documentation of accreditation for patient care. Remember that the site visitor can ask for additional materials to support institutional oversight and evidence of quality education, work environment, and patient care.

Good luck!

MASTER AFFILIATION AGREEMENT FOR MAJOR PARTICIPATING INSTITUTIONS

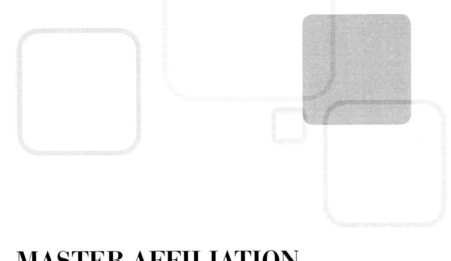

MASTER AFFILIATION AGREEMENT FOR MAJOR PARTICIPATING INSTITUTIONS

This master affiliation agreement for *major participating institutions* in which residents rotate ("Agreement") is between [Name of sponsoring institution] ("Sponsoring Institution") and [Name of major participating institution] ("Participating Institution").

Whereas, the Sponsoring Institution hosts medical education programs for residents and/or fellows, "physicians-in-training" who are in the Sponsoring Institution's graduate medical education (GME) programs for physicians;

Whereas, the term "physicians-in-training" means the Sponsoring Institution's residents and fellows;

Whereas, the Participating Institution in [City, State] desire to serve as a rotation facility for the program residents and/or fellows and the accreditation agencies require the Sponsoring Institution to be responsible for the quality of all educational experience and to retain authority over trainees' activities; and

Whereas, this Agreement will: (1) identify the officials at the Participating Institution who will assume administrative, educational, and supervisory responsibility for the trainees; (2) outline the educational goals and objectives

---

to be attained within the Participating Institution; (3) specify the method of assignment of the trainees to the Participating Institution; (4) determine the Participating Institution's responsibilities for teaching, supervising, and formally evaluating residents and fellows; and (5) establish with the Participating Institution the policies and procedures that govern the trainees' education while rotating at the Participating Institution.

Therefore, the Sponsoring Institution and Participating Institution hereby agree to establish a GME rotation upon the terms and conditions as follows:

A. **Resident rotation(s).** The parties shall establish a physicians-in-training rotation at the Participating Institution that will be affiliated with the GME programs at the Sponsoring Institution, and participation in the GME programs by the residents and fellows is acknowledged as a bona fide rotation for the GME programs. The Sponsoring Institution, through its program director and upon mutual agreement with the Participating Institution and its key administration, will recommend the number of interns or residents that will participate in each rotation. The parties agree that the participants, GME program descriptions, objectives, and specifications of each agreed upon rotation must be documented and signed by all parties as a separate addendum to this Agreement, or separate agreements, to be effective. See Program Letter of Agreement in Appendix 2 for examples of key components.

B. **Supervision of physicians-in-training.** The staff specialists assigned to provide training and supervision will be solely responsible for direct clinical supervision of the residents and fellows and shall control the details of the medical tasks performed by the physicians-in-training in compliance with accreditation agency standards and the Participating Institution's professional staff bylaws, manuals, rules, regulations, policies, and procedures. Residents and fellows will not be permitted to see patients at the Participating Institution unless the designated staff specialist is present to supervise or unless the residents are permitted to take call for a staff specialist under the terms of a specific written document from the program director noting standards for graduated patient care based on experience and training. Staff specialists shall be either employed physicians or other members of the active professional staff of the Participating Institution, who have agreed in writing to train and supervise interns, residents, and fellows.

C. **Qualifications of supervising physicians.** The staff specialists assigned to supervise the residents and fellows are subject to approval for participation in the rotation by the Sponsoring Institution's program director and the Participating Institution's key administrative leaders.

D. **Residents' and fellows' participation in care.** While rotating at the Participating Site, the residents and fellows may be involved in the care and treatment of patients only under the direction and supervision of the staff specialists assigned to provide training and supervision. The staff specialist shall have primary responsibility for the care of the patients, but may delegate patient care duties consistent with the policy of the hospital as related to resident training. The residents and fellows shall not have any primary, unsupervised patient care responsibility delegated to them by the staff specialists. The staff specialist is solely responsible for the patient care provided to the patients of the participating institution.

E. **Compliance with protocols.** All residents and fellows assigned to the participating institution under this Agreement will adhere to the bylaws, manuals, rules, regulations, and policies of the professional staff of the Participating Institution, and policies and procedures of the Sponsoring Institution and the department sponsoring the GME programs. Any physician-in-training failing to comply with the requirements in this paragraph may be terminated from participation in a specific GME program immediately. Both the Sponsoring Institution and the Participating Institution will make readily available to the residents and fellows all bylaws, manuals, rules, regulations, and policies of the professional staff and of the department, which are applicable to their participation in the rotation.

F. **Compliance with standards.** Residents and fellows rotating at the participating institution shall comply with the standards of both the Sponsoring Institution and the Participating Institution.

G. **Prerequisites.** The sponsoring institution will ensure that residents and fellows:

    1. Have received instruction in universal blood and body fluid precautions (within the past year) and cardiopulmonary resuscitation (a healthcare basic life support/CPR course within the past two years).

    2. Have all immunizations required by applicable regulatory agencies and the Participating Institution's policies, including hepatitis B (or waiver) and current purified protein derivative (PPD) test for tuberculosis, and provide evidence of immunity to chicken pox, measles, and rubella.

    3. Have been tested for tuberculosis within one year of starting at the Participating Institution, are tested at least annually while at the Participating Institution, and provide evidence of such testing and results to the Participating Institution as required.

4. Have been administered a drug test prior to assignment to the Participating Institution in accordance with the current community standards for drug testing and background screening, and shall provide the results of such screen to the Participating Institution in accordance with the institutional standards. Should the Participating Institution provide the test, the Sponsoring Institution will be responsible for the reasonable cost of the test and will pay for such prior to any testing.

5. Have a background evaluation, including a criminal background evaluation/history that is provided to the Participating Institution. Individuals who have been convicted of a crime, other than a misdemeanor driving violation, in the past seven years will not be permitted to participate in the program. Depending on the nature of the conviction, individuals with convictions more than seven years old may not be eligible to participate. Should the Participating Institution provide the background evaluation, the Sponsoring Institution will be responsible for the reasonable cost of the evaluation, and will pay for such prior to the evaluation.

6. Shall provide the Participating Institution with (a) an executed copy of the "Release from Liability," (b) written documentation of current health insurance, and (c) other written documentation as required by this agreement. Such documentation is to be submitted to the Medical Staff Services office in accordance with the Participating Institution's policy.

H. **Confidentiality of Patient Information.** All parties acknowledge the obligations of the Health Insurance Portability and Accountability Act of 1996 ("HIPAA") and other regulations implementing HIPAA (42 U.S.C. § 1320(d). The Sponsoring Institution will ensure that each resident and/or fellow agrees to maintain the confidentiality of individually identifiable health information of patients as required by HIPAA and as required by state law.

I. **Goals.** The rotation shall strive to achieve the goals and objectives established by the Sponsoring Institution's program director, which must be appended to this Agreement by a separate addendum, or separate agreement.

J. **Compensation.** Throughout the term of this Agreement, residents and fellows are employees of the Sponsoring Institution. Residents and fellows are responsible for all lodging, parking, and meals. Residents and fellows shall receive no monetary compensation, employee benefits, or other type of remuneration from the Participating Institution.

K. Liability Coverage. Residents and fellows shall be provided with professional liability coverage by the Sponsoring Institution (or the Participating Institution, as negotiated) through its liability indemnification protocols routinely used for its residents and fellows or in another manner of the institution's choosing. (Specify limits.)

L. Term and Termination. This Agreement shall remain in full force and effect for a term of one year beginning July 1, 200_, with automatic renewal annually up to a maximum of five years, unless the Agreement is terminated or canceled by either party.

1. *Termination without cause.* Either party upon [specify number of days] days' written notice may terminate this Agreement, any addendum, or separate agreement without cause.

2. *Termination for default.* Either party may terminate this Agreement effective immediately and without penalty if and when it determines in its sole discretion and judgment that the other party is not complying with the terms of this Agreement.

3. *Automatic termination.* In the event that the Participating Institution enters bankruptcy, takes an assignment for the benefit of creditors, becomes subject to receivership, or is otherwise reasonably deemed insolvent, this Agreement shall terminate at the option of the Sponsoring Institution.

M. Notice. Any notice to be given pursuant to this Agreement or any addendum shall be given to the respective parties in writing either by personal delivery or by registered or certified mail, postage prepaid, as follows:

Participating Institution:
Address
Name of responsible individual

Sponsoring Institution:
Address
Name of responsible individual

Such notice shall be deemed to have been given three days following deposit in the United States mail, unless actually received sooner by mail or personal delivery.

N. Miscellaneous. All parties agree to the following conditions:

1. *Use of name:* Advertising. Neither party shall use the other's name or any corporate or business name which is reasonably likely to suggest that the two parties are related, without first obtaining the written consent of the other party.

2. *Nonassignment and subcontracting.* The participating institution shall not assign, transfer, or contract for the furnishing of services to be performed under this Agreement without the prior written approval of the Sponsoring Institution.

3. *Entire agreement.* This Agreement and its addenda constitute the entire understanding between the parties with respect to the subject matter hereof and may be modified only by a written document signed by both parties.

4. *Severability.* In the event that one or more clauses of this Agreement are declared illegal, void, or unenforceable, that shall not affect the validity of the remaining portions of this Agreement.

5. *Waiver.* The failure of either party to exercise any of its rights under this Agreement for a breach thereof shall not be deemed to be a waiver of such rights, and no waiver by either party, whether written or oral, expressed or implied, of any rights under or arising from the Agreement shall be binding on any subsequent occasion, and no concession by either party shall be treated as an implied modification of the Agreement unless specifically agreed in writing.

6. *Nonexclusive.* This Agreement is not intended to be exclusive of any other arrangements between a party or parties to this Agreement, and any third party or parties. Each party hereto shall retain, without limitation, the right to enter into like or similar arrangements with the other parties hereto and/or any third party or parties.

Sponsoring Institution

[Name of Institution]

By: _____

      [Signature of designated official]

_____

      [Name/title of designated official]

Date: _____

Participating Institution

[Name of Institution]

By: _____

      [Signature of designated official]

_____

      [Name/title of designated official]

Date: _____

FIGURE A.1

Exhibit Examples

Examples of exhibits that may be attached to the master affiliation agreement include the following:

- Community standard for drug screening
- Criminal background checks
- Agreement for release of liability during rotation experience at the Participating Institution
- Acknowledgment of administrative, educational, and supervisory responsibility
- Program letter of agreements specifying responsibilities, goals and objectives, liability, and so forth
- Compensation arrangements
- Resident rotation schedules, including dates, rotations, and durations

PROGRAM LETTER OF AGREEMENT FOR ROTATIONS

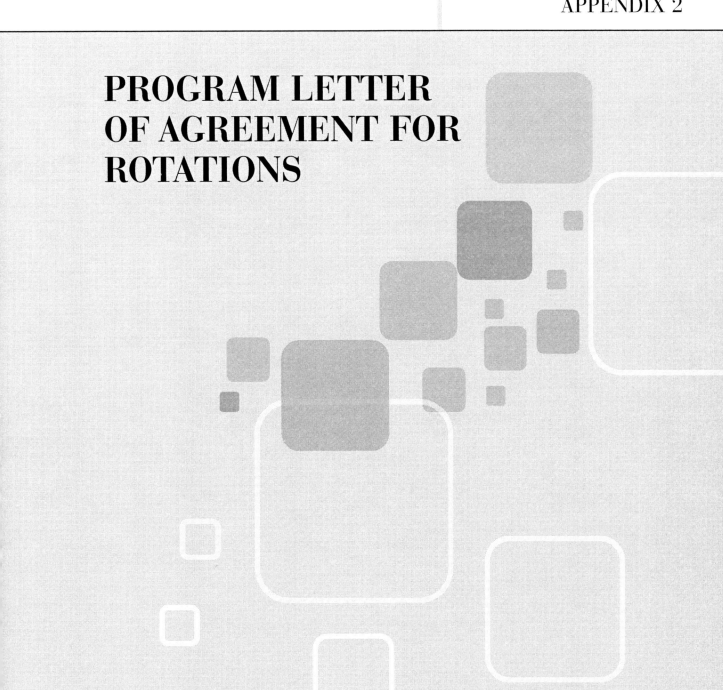

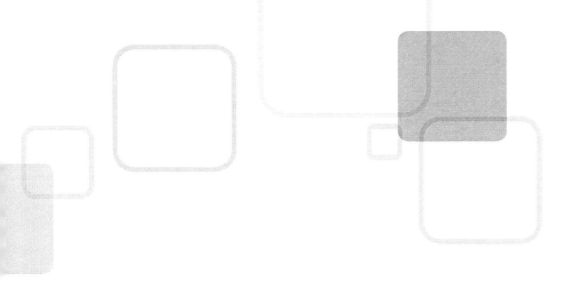

PROGRAM LETTER OF AGREEMENT FOR ROTATIONS

This program letter of agreement ("Agreement"), is made and entered into on this the __ day of _____, 200_, by and between [name of Sponsoring Institution, Department, and Program] ("Sponsoring Institution"), located at [address], and [name of Participating Site and Program] ("Participating Site") located at [address].

Whereas, the Sponsoring Institution, in furtherance of its statutory obligations to provide health care services to the residents of CITY, STATE, owns and operates a fully accredited, integrated health delivery system;*

Whereas, the Sponsoring Institution hosts education programs for physicians-in-training, who are in the Sponsoring Institution's [specialty] Residency or Fellowship Program ("Program");

Whereas, Participating Site is a medical center or outpatient facility providing treatment to the people of CITY, STATE, and surrounding areas and is desirous of the services of physicians-in-training in the Sponsoring Institution's Program;

Whereas, Participating Site desires to serve as a resident or fellow rotation facility for the Program resident(s) and/ or fellow(s) and the [name of accreditation agency] requires the Sponsoring Institution to be responsible for the quality of all educational experience and to retain authority over trainees' activities; and

Whereas, this agreement will: (1) identify the officials at the Participating Site who will assume administrative, educational, and supervisory responsibility for the residents; (2) outline the educational goals and objectives to be attained within the Participating Site; (3) specify the period of assignment of the residents to the Participating Site, the financial arrangements, and the details for insurance and benefits; (4) determine the Participating Site's responsibilities for teaching, supervising, and formally evaluating residents; and (5) establish with the Participating Site the policies and procedures that govern the residents' education while rotating to the Participating Site.*

I. Goals and Objectives

A. **Resident rotation.** The parties hereto shall establish a program resident rotation ("Rotation") at the Participating Site that will be affiliated with the Program at the Sponsoring Institution, and participation in said Program by the residents is acknowledged as a bona fide Rotation for the Program. The parties agree that the annual assignment of residents and the length of each assignment shall depend on the availability of such residents for assignments and the time allotted by the Program director to each resident for rotations.

B. **Supervision of residents.** The Participating Site staff specialists assigned to provide training and supervision will be responsible for direct clinical supervision of the residents while at the participating site and shall control the details of the medical tasks performed by the residents in compliance with accreditation standards and in keeping with the supervision policy of the Sponsoring Institution attached hereto and incorporated herein by reference. [Attach policy.]

C. **Qualifications of supervising physicians.** The staff specialists assigned to supervise the residents are subject to approval for participation in the rotation by the Sponsoring Institution's Program director. All physicians performing services pursuant to this Agreement shall possess all necessary qualifications, training, and experience as recommended by the Accreditation Council for Graduate Medical Education (ACGME), and, as applicable, current licensure or certification in the State.

D. **Resident participation in care.** While at the Participating Site, the residents may be involved in the care and treatment of patients only under the direction and supervision of the staff specialists assigned to provide training and supervision. The Participating Site staff specialist shall have primary responsibility for the care of patients, but may delegate patient care duties (e.g., rounds), as deemed appropriate, to the residents. The residents shall not have any primary, unsupervised patient care responsibility delegated to them by staff specialists as primary providers.

E. **Compliance with protocols.** Each resident assigned to the participating site under this Agreement will adhere to the bylaws, rules, regulations, and policies of the medical staff of the Participating Site, and to the policies of the Sponsoring Institution and the department sponsoring the Program. Any resident failing to comply with the above requirements may be terminated immediately.

F. **Compliance with standards.** The residents rotating at the Participating Site shall comply with the standards of the Participating Site and Sponsoring Institution.

G. **Liability coverage.** Residents shall be provided with professional liability coverage by the [Sponsoring Institution or Participating Site, as negotiated] through its liability indemnification protocols routinely used for its Resident physicians-in-training. [Specify limits.]

H. **Term and termination.** This Agreement shall remain in full force and effect for a term of one year beginning July 1, 200_, and expiring June 30, 200_, and shall automatically renew for successive one-year periods upon the Sponsoring Institution updating the list of Residents participating in the Rotation, unless the Agreement is terminated or canceled by either party. This Agreement and its renewals shall not exceed a total term of five years.

   1. *Termination without cause.* Either party upon [specify number of days] days written notice may terminate this agreement without cause.

   2. *Termination for default.* Either party may terminate this agreement effective immediately and without penalty if and when it determines, in its sole discretion and judgment, which the other party is not complying with terms of this agreement.

   3. *Automatic termination.* In the event that the Participating Site enters bankruptcy, takes an assignment for the benefit of creditors, becomes subject to receivership, or is otherwise reasonably deemed insolvent, then this Agreement shall terminate at the option of the Sponsoring Institution.

I. **Notices.** All notices provided for by this Agreement shall be made in writing either (1) by actual delivery (e.g., personally, by commercial courier service, or by confirmed facsimile) of the notice, or (2) by the mailing of the notice by United States Postal Service certified or registered mail, return receipt requested, and addressed to the party to be notified at the address set forth below (or at such other address as may be given by notice of a party). The notice shall be deemed to be received (a) if by actual delivery, on the date of its receipt by the party, or (b) if by mail, on the second day on which mail is delivered following the date of deposit in the United States Postal Service.

Participating Site	Sponsoring Institution
Name and title of responsible individual Address	Name and title of responsible individual Address

J. **Miscellaneous.** All parties agree to the following conditions:

1. *Use of name: Advertising.* Neither party shall use the other's name or any corporate or business name which is reasonably likely to suggest that the two parties are related, without first obtaining the written consent of the other party.

2. *Nonassignment and subcontracting.* Participating Site shall not assign, transfer, or contract for the furnishing of services to be performed under this Agreement without the written approval of Sponsoring Institution.

3. *Waiver.* The failure of either party to exercise any of its rights under this Agreement for a breach thereof shall not be deemed to be a waiver of such rights, and no waiver by either party, whether written or oral, expressed or implied, of any rights under or arising from the Agreement shall be binding on any subsequent occasion, and no concession by either party shall be treated as an implied modification of the Agreement unless specifically agreed in writing.

4. *Attorney's fees and court costs.* If either party brings an action against the other to enforce any condition or covenant of this Agreement, each party shall be individually responsible for its own court costs and attorney's fees.

5. *Binding agreement.* The parties hereto warrant and represent that upon execution hereof, this Agreement shall be a legal, valid, and binding obligation on them and shall be enforceable against them in accordance with its terms. The individuals signing this Agreement warrant and represent that they are duly authorized to sign this Agreement on behalf of the parties hereto.

Sponsoring Institution

[Name of Institution]

By: _____

        [Signature of designated official]

_____

        [Name/title of designated official]

Date: _____

Participating Institution

[Name of Institution]

By: _____

        [Signature of designated official]

_____

        [Name/title of designated official]

Date: _____

Key points in creating the program letter of agreement.

Note: Most programs only complete the PLA portion of this agreement. However, institutions may require a formal rotation agreement for each rotation outside of the sponsoring institution or a modified version of the rotation agreement. ACGME requires a PLA with key components as outlined.

Attachment 1

Program letter of agreement

A. Residency program:

B. Sponsoring institution:

C. Participating site:

D. Location and rotation:

E. Summary description:

F. Objectives:

G. Faculty:

1. List faculty appointed to supervise residents for this Rotation.

2. Responsibilities of faculty at Participating Site:
   a. Direct supervision of rotating residents
   b. Deliver medical education on rounds and in structured learning setting to meet ACGME competencies
   c. Ensure that learning activities meet the goals and objectives of the Rotation developed by the Program director at the Sponsoring Institution
   d. Evaluate residents using set standards and criteria from the Program director at the Sponsoring Institution to monitor the ACGME competencies
   e. Report evaluation results in a timely manner to Sponsoring Institution's Program director

H. Period of assignment:

Academic Year _____

Resident/Fellow	Post graduate year	Beginning date	Ending date

I. **Financial arrangements**

Attach financial arrangement schedule, including benefit and liability coverage as applicable.

J. **Additional policies and procedures**

Attach additional policies and procedures.